Biochemistry

By

Target Educare

Biochemistry

By
Target Educare

- Topic wise arranged MCQs of AIIMS & All India Postgraduate Entrance Exam. (with explanatory Answers)
- Also useful for 1st year students

Manisha Bansal

CBS PUBLISHERS & DISTRIBUTORS
NEW DELHI • BANGALORE (INDIA)

978-81-89253-78-6
ISBN : 978-81-239-1517-3

First Edition : 2007

Publishing Director : Vinod K. Jain

Published by :
Satish Kumar Jain for CBS Publishers & Distributors,
4596/1-A, 11 Darya Ganj, New Delhi - 110 002 (India)
E-mail: cbspubs@vsnl.com • Website: www.cbspd.com

Branch Office :
2975, 17th Cross, K.R. Road, Bansankari 2nd Stage, Bangalore-70
Fax : 080-26771680 • E-mail : cbsbng@vsnl.net

Composed by :
LineArt Graphics, Delhi-110091

Printed at :
Asia Printograph, Delhi

Preface

Biochemistry is a unique book providing adequate information on the subject in a concise manner. The striking feature of the book is its attention to details that are asked in various multiple choice examinations.

The chapters begin with a brief synopsis of the topic, followed by multiple choice questions with explanatory answers. A question bank has been added at the end for the benefit of students for self assessment and review.

Recent syllabus, repeated questions and vital topics have all been taken into consideration during the preparation of the manuscript.

Readers are requested to communicate their views for the further improvement of the book in future.

Wish you all the very best

AUTHORS

Contents

1

Cell Biology

1. Cell is defined as: Structural and functional unit of life.
2. Major components of cell membrane: Lipids (Phospholipids, Glycolipids, Cholesterol) and Proteins (Integral proteins, Peripheral proteins)
3. Major phospholipids of cell membrane: Glycerophospholipids.
4. Cholesterol forms: The central hydrophobic layer in the membrane.
5. The fluidity of the membrane is controlled by: Cholesterol.
6. The fluidity of cell membrane increases with: Increase in unsaturated fatty acids.
7. Membrane proteins are mostly: Glycoproteins.
8. The entire outer surface of the cell often has a loose carbohydrate coat called as: Glycocalyx.
9. Nucleolus is an accumulation of large amounts of RNA and proteins inside the: Nucleus.
10. The artificial products of intracellular membranes derived from endoplasmic reticulum are called as: Microsomes.
11. Majority of mitochondrial proteins are synthesized: Outside mitochondria in free polyribosomes.
12. The most important function of the golgi apparatus is: The post- translational modification of primitive proteins.
13. Lysosomes are richly contain: Hydrolases.
14. Characteristic feature of lysosomal hydrolases: They contain mannose 6-phosphate and have optimum pH = 4 - 5.
15. Peroxisomes contain the enzymes: Peroxidases and catalases
16. Absense of peroxisomes causes an inherited disorder called as: Zellweger's Syndrome.
17. Cytoskeleton consist of: Microfilaments; intermediate filaments: Microtubules.
18. The intermediate filament having highest molecular weight: Neurofilaments.
19. The fluidity of cell membrane increases with increase in: Unsaturated fatty acid.

	Organelle	Marker	Major Functions
1.	Nucleus	DNA	Site of chromosomes, Site of DNA-directed RNA synthesis.
2.	Mitochondiria	Glutamic dehydrogenase	Citric acid cycle, oxidative phosphorylation.
3.	Ribosome	High content of RNA	Site of protein synthesis.
4.	ER	Glucose-6-phosphatase	Membranes-bound ribosome is a major site of protein synthesis–Synthesis of various lipids -Oxidation of many xenobiotics.
5.	Lysosome	Acid phosphatase	-Site of many hydrolases involved in catalyzing degradative reactions.
6.	Plasma membrane	Na-K-ATPase and 5'-nucleotidase	-Transport of molecules in and out of cells. Intercellular adhesion and communication.
7.	Golgi Apparatus	Galactosyl transferase	-Intracellular sorting of proteins. Glycosylation reactions. Sulfating reactions.
8.	Peroxisomes	Catalase Uric acid oxidase	-Degradation of certain fatty acids and amino acids. Production and degradation of hydrogen peroxide.

PLASMA PROTEINS

1. Plasma is the liquid medium of blood constituting about: 55-60% of blood.
2. A liquid medium from blood with an anticoagulant is: Plasma.
3. A liquid medium from blood without an anticoagulant is: Serum (defibrinated plasma).
4. Total protein content of normal plasma is: 6-8 gm/100 ml.
5. Plasma proteins are synthesized in cell in: Membrane bound polyribosome.
6. Majority of plasma proteins are glycoprotein, except: Albumin.
7. Plasma proteins are mostly synthesized in: Liver.
8. Commonly employed method for seperation of plasma proteins is: Electrophoresis.
9. Almost all proteins in the blood function as: Transport proteins for hydrophobic substances.
10. Plasma proteins are separated as: Albumin and globulins.
11. 5 different types of globulins can be separated out as: á$_1$, á$_2$, â$_1$, â$_2$and ã-globulins.
12. Each type of globulin again includes: Different protein with different chemical nature.
13. Major serine protease inhibitor in plasma is: á$_1$ – antitrypsin.
14. The most important platelet activator is: Thrombin.
15. The thrombolytic agent having selectivity for fibrin clot is: Plasmin.
16. A mucopolysaccharide that terminates clot formation by interfering with a number of steps in the coagulation cascade is: Heparin.
17. The first class of antibodies to be observed in the plasma following antigenic stimulation: IgM.

18. A glycopeptide molecule which helps in polymerization of IgA and IgM monomer is: J chain.
19. Light chain proteins, insoluble at boiling point and precipitated at 60°C, found in urine in multiple myeloma: Bence-Jones protein.
20. Light chain fragments of globulins in urine are called as: Bence Jones protein.

HUMAN IMMUNOLOBULINS					
	IgG	IgA	IgM	IgD	IgE
Heavy chains	ã	α	μ	δ	ε
Light chains	λ	λ	λ	λ	λ
Molecular weight	150,000	170,000	960,000	184,000	188,100
Normal serum concentration	8.16 g/l	1.4 – 4	0.5 – 2.0	0 – 0.4	0.1 – 1.3
Ability to cross placenta	Yes	No	No	No	No

SOLVED QUESTIONS

Q.1. Membrane fluidity is increased by: (AIIMS MAY 2005)

1. **Stearic acid**
2. **Palmitic acid**
3. **Cholesterol**
4. **Linoleic acid**

Ans. 4

The lipid bilayer shows free lateral movement of its components, hence the membrane is said to be fluid in nature. Fluidity enables the membrane to perform endocytosis and exocytosis. The cholesterol content of the membrane alters the fluidity of the membrane. When cholesterol concentration increases, the membrane becomes less fluid on the outer surface, but more fluid in the hydrophobic core. The nature of fatty acids also affects the fluidity of the membrane, the more unsaturated cis fatty acids increase the fluidity.

Q.2. The transmembrane region of protein is likely to have: (AIPGME 2004)

1. **A stretch of hydrophilic amino acids**
2. **A stretch of hydrophobic amino acids**
3. **A disulphide loop**
4. **Alternating hydrophilic and hydrophobic amino acids**

Ans. 2

Proteins present in cell membrane are amphipathic and form an integral part of the membrane by having hydrophilic regions protruding at the inside and outside faces of the membrane but connected by a hydrophobic region traversing the hydrophobic core of the bilayer. Those portions of membrane proteins that traverse membranes do contain substantial numbers of hydrophobic amino acids.

Q.3. In dividing cells, spindle is formed by: **(AIPGME 2002)**

1. **Ubiquitin**
2. **Tubulin**
3. **Laminin**
4. **Keratin**

Ans. 2

Tubulin – Microtubules an integral component of the cellular cytoskeleton, are necessary for the formation and function of mitotic spindles and thus are present in all eukaryotic cells. Microtubules are cylinders of 13 longitudinally arranged protofilaments, each consisting of dimers of á-tubulin and â-tubulin.

Ubiquitin – It targets many intracellular proteins for degradation. It is a small protein (8.5 kDa) present in all eukaryotic cells.

Laminin – It is a basement membrane protein component of renal, glomerular and other basal laminae.

Keratin – It is a structural protein present in hairs and nails.

Q.4. The cellular component for protein synthesis is: **(AIPGME 1997)**

1. **Smooth endoplsmic reticulum**
2. **Rough endoplasmic reticulum**
3. **Ribosomes**
4. **Mitochondria**

Ans. 3

Protein synthesis takes place on ribosomes that are bound to endoplasmic reticulum or cytosolic or mitochondiral ribosomes.

Q.5. A marker of golgi apparatus is: **(AIPGME 1995)**

1. **Galactosyl transferase**
2. **Acetyl CoA synthetase**
3. **Pyruvate kinase**
4. **Malonyl CoA**

Ans. 1

Some enzymes are present in certain organelles only; Such specific enzymes are called as marker enzymes. Galactosyl transferase is the marker of golgi- apparatus. The carbohydrate chains are added to newly synthesised protein molecules in the golgi bodies with the help of this enzyme. Acetyl CoA synthetase, pyruvate kinase and malonyl CoA are not specific markers for any sub-cellular organelles.

Examples of some specific markers:

Organelle	Marker
1. Nucleus	DNA
2. Mitochondria	Glutamic dehydrogenase
3. Ribosome	RNA
4. Endoplasmic reticulum	Glucose -6- phosphatase
5. Lysosome	Acid phosphatase
6. Peroxisome	Catalase

Q.6. Cell shape and motility are provided by: **(AIPGME 1995)**

1. **Microfilaments**
2. **Microtubules**
3. **Golgi apparatus**
4. **Mitochondria**

Ans. 2

Microtubules, an integral component of the cellular cytoskeleton is involved in the intracellular movement of endocytic and exocytic vesicles and form the major structural components of cilia and flagella. They are also necessary for formation and function of the mitotic spindle.Microfilaments. (actin filaments) in nonmuscle cells interact with myosin to cause cellular movements. Golgi – apparatus and mitochondria are intracellular organelles. Golgi apparatus functions in glycosylation of proteins. ATP generation reactions and TCA cycle are related with mitochondria.

Q.7. Catabolism of H_2O_2 is carried out by: **(AIPGME 1994)**

1. **Peroxisomes**
2. **Mitochondria**
3. **Endoplasmic reticulum**
4. **Lysosomes**

Ans. 1

Peroxidation of polyunsaturated fatty acids in vivo may lead to hydroperoxide formation. Peroxisomes contain catalase and peroxidase which destroys the H_2O_2. Mitochondria is related with electron transport chain, ATP generation, TCA, cycle, different pathways of lipid metabolism etc. Rough endoplasmic reticulum is the site of protein biosynthesis. Lysosomes contain polysaccharide, protein, lipid, and nucleic acid hydrolysing enzymes.Thus only peroxisomes contain the enzyme necessary to split H_2O_2.

Q.8. Which biochemical reaction does not occurs in the mitochondria: **(AIPGME 1994)**

1. **Kreb's cycle**
2. **Urea cycle**
3. **Gluconeogenesis**
4. **Fatty acid synthesis**

Ans. **4**

The enzymes for fatty acid synthesis are located in the cytosol-only. Kerb's cycle occurs in mitochondrial matrix. Some steps of urea cycle occur in mitochondria while some in cytosol. In case of gluconeogenesis also first reaction takes place in mitochondria and rest in cytosol.

Q.9. Which one of the following amino acids is most likely to be found in the transmembrane region of a protein: (AIIMS Nov. 2005)

1. **Lysine**
2. **Arginine**
3. **Leucine**
4. **Aspartate**

Ans. **3**

The transmembrane region of protein contain hydrophobic amino acids as this region contains hydrophobic lipids. Among the above mentioned amino acids, leucine is the one having hydrophobic nature. Lysine, arginine and aspartate are hydrophilic in nature.

Q.10. RBC membrane is maintained by: (AIIMS May 2002)

1. **Spectrin**
2. **Laminin**
3. **Collagen**
4. **Elastin**

Ans. **1**

Cytoskeleton is responsible for the shape of the cell. RBC cytoskeleton contains spectrin, a tetramer composed of alpha and beta polypeptides. Laminin is a basement membrane protein with adhesive properties that enable epithelial cell to fix to underlying connective tissue. Collagen and elastin are structural proteins found in connective tissue.

Q.11. Which of these is not a part of extracellular matrix: (AIIMS May 2002)

1. **Laminin**
2. **Fibronectin**
3. **Integrins**
4. **Collagen**

Ans. **3**

Most mammalian cells are located in tissue where they are surrounded by a complex extracellular matrix, often referred to as "connective tissue". The extracellular matrix contain three major classes of biomolecules:

1. The structural proteins – Collagen, Elastin and Fibrillin.
2. Certain specialised proteins – Fibrillin, Fibronectin and Laminin.
3. Proteoglycans.

Integrins-are adhesive proteins located on the surface of neutrophils. They are involved in the adhesion of cells to other cells or to specific components of the extracellular matrix.

Q.12. Which of the following membrane has the highest protein content per gram tissue: (AIIMS May 2002)

1. **Inner mitochondrial membrane**
2. **Outer mitochondrial membrane**
3. **Plasma membrane**
4. **Myelin sheath**

Ans. 1

Composition of cell membrane (by weight)

Membrane	Protein %	Llipid %	Carbohydrate %
Myelin	20	75	05
Erythrocyte	49	43	08
Hepatocyte plasma membrane	54	39	07
Outer mitochondrial membrane	50	46	04
Inner mitochondrial membrane	75	23	02

Q.13. Which of the following dose not cross the cell membrane: (AIIMS May 2002)

1. **Glucose-6-phosphate**
2. **Glucose**
3. **Nitrous oxide**
4. **Carbon monoxide**

Ans. 1

In the cell membrane specific transporters for glucose are present. There are no such transporters for glucose-6-phosphate. To cross the cell membrane glucose-6-phosphate should be converted to glucose by the enzyme glucose-6-phosphatase.

Q.14. Receptor mediated endocytosis is by: (AIIMS Dec. 1998)

1. **Clathrin**
2. **Porine**
3. **Cytocin**
4. **Vimentin.**

Ans. 1

Two types of endocytosis: An endocytic vesicle forms as a result of invagination of a portion of the plasma membrane. Fluid phase endocytosis is random and nondirected. Receptor mediated endocytosis is selective and occurs in coated pits lined with the protein clathrin. Targeting is provided by receptors specific for a variety of molecules.

Q.15. Addition of PUFA in plasma membrane causes: (AIIMS June 1999)

1. **Membrane becomes rigid**
2. **Increase in fluidity of membrane**
3. **Decrease in fluidity of membrane**
4. **Nochange in fluidity of membrane**

Ans. 2

(Explanation same as Q. 1)

Q.16. Transition temperature of lipid bilayers of cell membrane is increased by: (AIIMS May 2001)

1. **Cholesterol**
2. **Saturated fatty acids**
3. **Hydrocarbons**
4. **Unsaturated fatty acids**

Ans. 2

The fluidity of membranes are largely dependent upon the lipid composition of the membrane.In a lipid bilayer, the hydrophobic chains of the fatty acids can be highly aligned or ordered to provide a rather stiff structures. As the temperature increases,the hydrophobic side chains undergo a transition from the ordered state (more gel-like or crystalline phase) to a disordered one, taking on a more liquid like or fluid arrangements. The temperature at which the structure undergoes the transition from ordered to disordered (i.e melts) is called the transition temperature.

The longer and more saturated fatty acid chains interact more strongly with each other via their longer hydrocarbon chains and thus cause higher values of Tm – i.e higher temperatures are required to increase the fluidity of the bilayer. On the other hand, unsaturated bonds that exist in the cis configuration tend to increase the fluidity of the bilayer. On the other hand, unsaturated bonds that exist in the cis configuration tend to increase the fluidity of a bilayer by decreasing the compactness of the side chain packing without diminishing hydrophobicity.

Q,17. The most abundant glycoprotein present in basement membrane is:

1. **Laminin**
2. **Fibronectin**
3. **Collagen type 4**
4. **Heparan sulphate.**

Ans. 1

Laminin: Is a glycoprotein with three polypeptide chains.It is a basement membrane protein with adhesive properties that enables epithelial cells to fix to underlying connective tissue.

Fibronectin: Is a cells surface protein that is involved in the interaction of cells with the extracellular matrix.

Collagen type IV: Is a structural protein in connective tissue. It is the major fibrous element of tissues.

Heparan sulphate: Is a mucopolysaccharide (glycosaminoglycan)

Q.18. Mitochondria is involved in all of the following except:

1. **ATP production**
2. **Apoptosis**
3. **TCA cycle**
4. **Fatty acid biosynthesis.**

Ans. 4

The enzymes for fatty acid biosynthesis are located in the cytosol only. ATP production (Electron transport chain) occurs on the inner surface of inner mitochondrial membrane. Enzymes for TCA cycle are located in mitochondrial matrix.Mitochondria are the control centers for regulating apoptosis (Programmed cell death).When mitochondria are damaged, mitochondrial permeability transition complex is opened and cytochrome C is liberated. This starts the caspase activation pathway, leading to cell death.

Q.19. DNA is found principally in:

1. **A Nucleolus**
2. **The Nucleus**
3. **The Cytoplasm**
4. **The Mitochondria.**

Ans. 2

Nucleus contains the DNA, the chemical basis of genes which governs all the functions of the cells. Nucleolus is the area for RNA processing and ribosome synthesis. Mitochondria are the power-house of the cell. In the cytoplasm the enzymes of various metabolic pathways like protein synthesis, glycolysis, glycogen metabolism etc are located.

Q.20. Which of the following about biological membrane is true:

1. **Lipid moiety is amphipathic**
2. **Rigid assembly of protein, lipid and carbohydrate**
3. **Symmetrical bi leaflet structures**
4. **Lipid and protein moiety are held by covalent interactions.**

Ans. 1

Bilayers, are the key structures in biological membranes. A bilayer exists as a sheet in which the hydrophobic regions of the phospholipids are protected from the aqueous environment, while the hydrophillic regions are immersed in water that means they are amphipathic in nature. Lipid bilayers are formed by self-assembly, driven by the hydrophobic effects.

Q.21. Agranular endoplasmic reticulum is involved in the synthesis of: (AIIMS Nov 2006)

1. **Protein.**
2. **Lipid.**
3. **Carbohydrate.**
4. **Vitamin D.**

Ans. 1

Due to the presence or absence of ribosomes endoplasmic reticulum are of two types: -

(a) Granular (ribosomes are present).

(b) Agranular (ribosomes are absent).

Due to the presence of ribosomes granular endoplasmic reticulum is involved in the synthesis of proteins. Where as agranular endoplasmic reticulum is involved in the synthesis of lipids, steroids and in the detoxification of drugs with the help of the enzyme Cytochrome p450.

Q.22. During phagocytosis, the metabolic process called respiratory burst involves the activation of: (AIPGEE 2006)

1. **Oxidase.**
2. **Hydrolase.**
3. **Peroxidase.**
4. **Dehydrogenase.**

Ans. 1

Phagocytosis is the process of engulfment and killing of bacteria by macrophages. It is accompanied by rapid consumption of O_2 and generation of free radicals CO_2, H_2O, HOCl and the reaction is carried out by NADPH oxidase. This process is reffered to as respiratory burst. Infact, the free radicals generated during respiratory burst kill bacteria. This is truly a beneficial affect of free radicals.

Q.23. Agranular ER produces/synthesizes? (AIPGEE 2007)

1. **Proteins.**
2. **Lipids.**
3. **Vitamins.**
4. **Carbohydraytes.**

Ans. 2

A large portion of the endoplasmic reticulum is studded with ribosomes to give a granular appearance, which is reffered to as rough ER. Ribosomes are the factories of protein synthesis. The smooth ER does not contain ribosomes. It is involved in the synthesis of lipids. (Triacylglycerols, phospholipids, sterols) and metabolism of drugs, besides supplying Ca^{2+} for the cellular fractions.

2

Carbohydrate

CHEMISTRY OF CARBOHYDRATES

1. Carbohydrates are defined as: Polyhydroxy aldehydes or ketones or substances that yield such compounds on hydrolysis.
2. Monosaccharides are: Simple carbohydrates having only one actual or potential sugar group. They can not be further hydrolysed.
3. Asymmetric carbon atom: A carbon atom to which four different atoms or groups of atoms are attached.
4. All carbohydrates have atleast one asymmetric carbon atom except: Dihydroxy acetone.
5. The number of asymmetric carbon atoms in glucose is: 4.
6. Stereoisomers: Compounds which have same structural formula but differ in spatial configuration. Number of possible isomers depends on number of asymmetric carbon atoms.
7. The number of stereoisomers of glucose can be: $2^4 = 16$.
8. The reference carbohydrate is: Glyceraldehyde.
9. D and L isomers are based on: Spatial arrangements of -H and -OH groups around the carbon atom just adjacent to the terminal primary alcohol carbon.
   (*a*) If -OH group on this carbon is towards right: D-isomer
   (*b*) If -OH group on this carbon is towards left: L-isomer
10. Epimers of glucose which differ from glucose in the orientation of -H and -OH group around a single carbon atom (other than the reference carbon atom) are – Mannose (2nd carbon), Galactose (4th carbon).
11. Dextrorotatory or D isomer – Rotate plane polarised light towards right.
    Levorotatory or L isomer – Rotate plane polarised light towards left.
12. Anomeric forms of glucose are: ∝-glucose and β-glucose
13. ∝-Anomer: -OH group on the anomeric carbon is below the plane of the ring.
    β-Anomer: -OH group on the anomeric carbon is above the plane of the ring.
14. Glucose molecule can be present as:- Straight chain
    Ring form Pyranose (6 membered), Furanose (5 membered).

15. Most of the glucose molecules are in: Pyranose ring form.
16. Fructose can be differentiated from glucose by: Seliwanoff's test and rapid furfural test.
17. Tests that detect the presence of reducing sugars are: Fehling's test, Benedict's test, Nylander's test.
18. Tests that differentiates monosaccharides from reducing disaccharides is: Barfoed's test given positive by monosaccharides only.
19. Benedict's test is a semiquantitative test, commonly employed to detect the presence of glucose in urine.
20. Specific method for blood glucose estimation is: Glucose oxidase peroxidase. It measures true glucose.
21. The disaccharides lactose, maltose and sucrose are respectively made of:

    Glucose + galactose (β-1, 4 linkage)

    Glucose + glucose (∝- 1, 4 linkage)

    Glucose + fructose (∝-1'→ β – 2 linkage).
22. Osazones of glucose and fructose – Broom shaped

    Osazones of maltose – Sunflower shaped

    Osazones of lactose – Powder puff shaped
23. Disaccharides that do not give the reducing tests for sugars are: Sucrose and trehalose.
24. Polysaccharides on hydrolysis yield: More than 10 monosaccharide units.
25. Homopolysaccharides of glucose with an:

    a.Unbranched structure is: Cellulose

    b.Branched structures are: Starch, glycogen and dextran.
26. Homopolysaccharide of fructose used for measuring GFR is: Inulin.
27. Homopolysaccharide of galactose: Agar.
28. Glycoproteins and proteoglycans are respectively: Branched chain and unbranched hetero-polysaccharides.
29. Glycoproteins consist of proteins covalently linked to: Oligosaccharide chains.
30. Carbohydrate content of mucoproteins is: > 10 %.

    Carbohydrate content of glycoproteins is: < 10 % .
31. Based on the linkage between the sugar and aminoacid, glycoproteins are classified as: N linked, O linked, GPI linked.
31. Mucins are rich in: O – linked glycoproteins.
32. ABO Blood group antigens are glycoproteins and contain the deoxy sugar: L-fucose.
33. Proteoglycans are proteins with covalently linked: Glycosaminoglycans.
34. Constituents of glycosaminoglycans are: Amino sugars and uronic acid.

35. The only glycosaminoglycan that dose not contain uronic acid is: Keratan sulfate.
36. Glycosaminoglycan molecules are: Polyanionic.
37. Function of glycoproteins is: Recognition sites on cell surfaces.

TABLE: 1 Classification of Monosaccharides

No. of Carbon atoms	Generic Name	Aldoses	Ketosugars
3	Triose	Glyceraldehyde	Dihydroxyacetone
4	Tetrose	Erythrose	Erythrulose
5	Pentose	Ribose, Xylose, Arabinose	Ribulose, Xylulose
6	Hexose	Glucose, Galactose, Mannose	Fructose
7	Heptose	Glucoheptose	Sedoheptulose

TABLE: 2 Structure and Occurrence of Glycosaminoglycans

Glycosaminoglycan	Repeating unit	Location
Hyaluronic acid	Glucuronic acid - N - acetylglucosamine	Joint fluid, vitreous humor
Chondroitin sulphate	Glucuronic acid - N - acetylgalactosamine*	Cartilage, bone, cornea
Keratan sulphate I	Galactose - N- acetylgalactosamine*	Cornea
Keratan sulphate II	Galactose - N- acetylgalactosamine*	Loose connective tissue
Heparin	Glucosamine*- L- iduronic acid	Mast cells
Heparan sulphate	Glucosamine - Glucuronic acid*	Skin, fibroblast, aortic walls
Dermatan sulphate	N-acetylgalactosamine*-L-iduronic acid*	Wide distribution

* -Indicates that the sugar is sulphated.

TABLE: 3 Mucoplysaccharidoses

Type	Syndrome	Enzyme Defect	Accumulated metabolite
I	Hurler	α-L-Iduronidase	Dermatan sulphate, heparan sulphate
II	Hunter	Iduronate sulfatase	Dermatan sulfate, heparan sulfate
III A	Sanfilippo A	Heparan sulfatase	Heparan sulfate
III B	Sanfilippo B	N-acetylglucosaminidase	Heparan sulfate
IV	Morquio	N-acetyl galactosamine-6-sulfatase	Keratan sulfate
VI	Maroteaux-lamy	N-actylgalactosamine-4-sulfatase	Dermatan sulfate
VII	Sly	β-Glucuronidase	Heparan sulfate

Glycolysis (Embden Meyerhoff Parnas Pathway)

1. It is the only pathway that is taking place in all the cells of the body.

2. Tissues dependent on glycolysis: Erythrocytes, cornea, lens and regions of retina, kidney medulla, testis, leucocytes.
3. Site of glycolysis: Cytosol.
4. Sources of carbon for glycolysis: Dietary starch, glycogen, sucrose, lactose, fructose.
5. Irreversible reactions are:

   (*a*) Glucose $\xrightarrow{\text{Hexokinase}}$ Glucose-6-phosphate.

   (*b*) Fructose-6-phosphate $\xrightarrow{\text{Phosphofructokinase}}$ Fructose 1, 6-bisphosphate.

   (*c*) Phosphoenol pyruvate $\xrightarrow{\text{Pyruvate kinase}}$ Pyruvate.
6. Site of hexokinase: All tissues except liver.

   Site of glucokinase: Only in liver.
7. Hexokinases differs from glucokinase in having: Low Km value for glucose.
8. Rate limiting enzyme in glycolysis is: Phosphofructokinase.
9. First committed step in glycolytic process is: Conversion of fructose-6-phosphate to fructose-1,6-bisphosphate by phosphofructokinase.
10. Activators of Phosphofructokinase (PFK): AMP, fructose-6-phosphate, fructose 2, 6-bisphosphate.

    Inhibitors of PFK: ATP, citrate.
11. Sodium fluoride used for blood glucose estimation inhibits the enzyme: Enolase.
12. Activators of pyruvate kinase:- Fructose 1,6,-bisphosphate,

    Inhibitors of pyruvate kinase:- ATP, alanine and acetyl COA.
13. Substrate level phosphorylation steps:

    (a) 1,3, bis phosphoglycerate $\xrightarrow{\text{Phosphoglycerate kinase}}$ 3-phosphoglycerate

    (b) Phosphoenol pyruvate $\xrightarrow{\text{Pyruvate kinase}}$ Pyruvate.
14. The overall reaction in glycolysis is:

    Glucose + 2 Pi + 2 ADP $\longrightarrow$ 2 Lactate + 2 ATP + 2 H_2O.
15. Total number of ATP's produced from 1 molecule of glucose under anaerobic conditions are: 2.
16. Total number of ATP's produced from 1 molecule of glucose under aerobic conditions are: 38.
17. Diversion in glycolytic pathway in erythrocytes is: Rapaport-Leubering Cycle [Bio-Phospho glycerate (BPG)-shunt].
18. Cells freely permeable to glucose are: Liver cells, pancreatic cells.
19. Pasteur effect states that: Under aerobic condition glycolysis is inhibited.
20. Crabtree effect states that: When oxygen supply is kept constant and glucose concentration is increased, comparative anaerobiosis is produced.

21. Disorders associated with impaired glycolysis:
    (a) Pyruvate kinase deficiency-Hemolytic anemia
    (b) Hexokinase deficiency–Reduces amount of oxygen that is available for tissues. Deficiency of this enzyme leads to low concentration of 1,3, BPG which is precursor of 2, 3-BPG. Thus low levels of 2, 3-BPG increases affinity of hemoglobin (Hb) for oxygen, oxygen saturation curve is shifted to left.
22. Hormones regulating glycolysis: Insulin favours glycolysis by activating key glycolytic enzymes. Glucocorticoids inhibit glycolysis.

Citric Acid cycle (Kreb's cycle or TCA cycle)

1. Location of the cycle: Mitochondrial matrix.
2. Final common pathway for oxidation of all major food stuffs is: Citric acid cycle.
3. Pyruvate dehydrogenase complex has: 3 enzymes:
   (a) Pyruvate dehydrogenase
   (b) Dihydrolipoyl transacetylase
   (c) Dihydrolipoyl dehydrogenase and 5 coenzymes – Thiamine pyrophosphate, lipoamide, coenzyme A, FAD and NAD.
4. Regulation of Pyruvate dehydrogenase (PDH) allosterically inhibited by acetyl COA, NADH and ATP. Insulin activates PDH.
5. Pyruvate as a junction point:
   (a) Decarboxylated to acetyl COA which enters the TCA cycle or may be utilized for fatty acid synthesis
   (b) Carboxylated to oxaloacetate which is used for gluconeogenesis
   (c) Transaminated to alanine.
6. Enzymes catalysing irreversible reactions of the TCA cycle are: Citrate synthase, α-ketoglutarate dehydrogenase.
7. Enzyme at substrate level phosphorylation step is: Succinate thiokinase.
8. Number of ATP produced in each TCA cycle: 12 ATP.
9. Number of CO_2 molecules formed in each TCA cycle: 2 molecules.
10. Fat can not be converted to glucose because: PDH reaction is an absolutely irreversible step.
11. Stoichiometry of TCA cycle:
    Acetyl COA + Oxaloacetate + FAD + 3 NAD^+ + GDP + Pi $\longrightarrow$ $2CO_2$ + CoA – SH + Oxaloacetate + $FADH_2$ + 3 NADH + GTP
12. The only amphibolic pathway is: TCA cycle

CITRIC ACID CYCLE

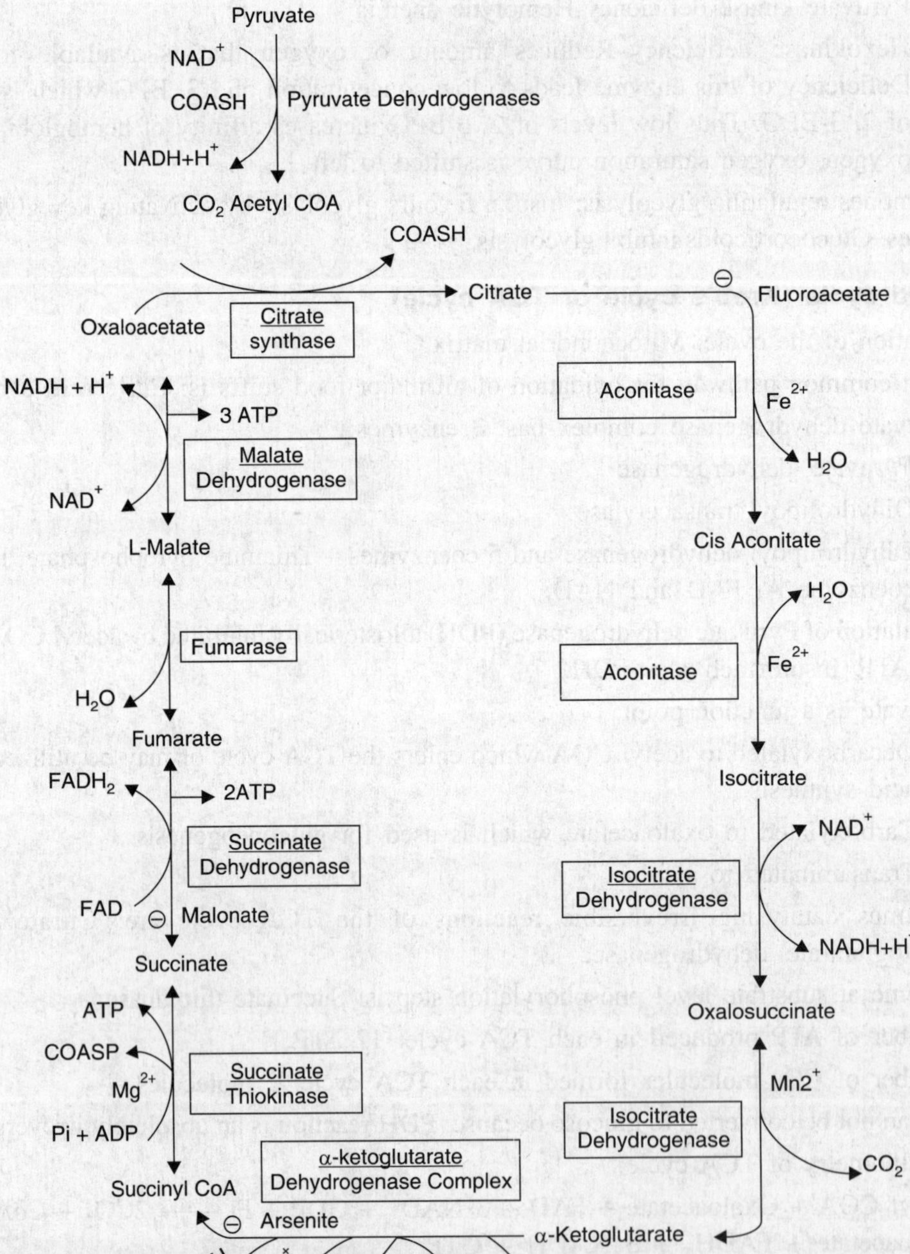

TABLE: Glycogen storage diseases

Type	Name Enzyme	Deficient	Inheritance Glycogen	Structure of Affected	Organs Clinical Features
1. Von Gierk's Disease	G-6-pase	Autosomal recessive	Normal (Metabollically NOT avilable)	Liver,Kidney, Intestine	Hypoglycaemia,s and Acidsis L.A,↑ Uric Acid ↑ Failure to thrive, Hepatomegaly
2. Pompe's Disease	Acid Maltase(Present in Lysosomes Catalyzes breakdown of oligosaccharides)	Autosomal recessive	Normal	Liver,Heart, Smooth and Straited muscles	Cardiomegaly, Muscle hypotonia No Hypoglycaemia
Note: Infants die of cardiac failure and bronchopneumonia. Death uaually before 9 months. A few survive 2½ years					
3. Limit Dextrinosis (Forbe's Disease)	Debranching enzyme	Autosomal recessive	Abnormal,'Limit Dextrin' type short missing outer branches	Liver (18%), Heart and Muscle (6%)	Moderate Hypoglycaemia Acidosis, Progressive myopathy, Hepatomegaly
Note: Patiants survive well to adult life					
4. Amylopectin--osis (Andersen's Disease)	Branching enzyme	Not known	Abnormal ("Amylopectin" type) Very long inner and outer unbranched chains, very few branch point	Liver, Heart, Muscle R.E system	Moderate hypoglycaemia Hepato-Splenomegaly, Ascites, Nodular Cirrhosis of Liver, Hepatic failure
Note: Prognosis fatal, longest survival reported as 4 years					
5. Mac Ardle's Disease	Muscle Phosphorylase	Autosomal recessive	Normal	Skeletal muscle (Excess normal glycogen Muscles)	Muscle cramps on exercise , Pian in muscle,weakness and Stiffness of muscle
Note: Affected children and adult, Muscle recovers with rest. Due to utilisation of F.A.for energy, after inj.epinephrine\) glucagon blood sugar (show Liver Phosphorylase not affected					
6. Her's Disease	Liver Phosphorylase	Autosomal Dominant	Normal	Liver, Leucocytes	Hypoglycaemia, Mild to moderate acidosis, Hepatomegaly
7. Tarui's Disease	Phosphofructokinase	--	--	--	As in type V
8. Hepatic Phosphorylase Kinase	Liver Phosphorylase Kinase		--	--	As in type VI

Hexose Monophosphate shunt (Pentose Phosphate Pathway)

1. Synonyms of pathway: Phosphogluconate oxidative pathway, Dickens- Horecker pathway.
2. Location of the pathway: Cytosol.
3. The pathway operates in following tissues: RBC, adrenal cortex, liver, testis, ovary, lactating mammary gland , and lens and cornea of eye.
4. The pathway is not seen in: Non lactating mammary gland.
5. Two phases of HMP shunt pathway are: Oxidative irreversible phase and Non-oxidative reversible phase.
6. Rate limiting enzyme of the pathway is: Glucose -6- phosphate dehydrogenase.
7. Regulation of HMP shunt: High level of NADPH inhibits glucose–6–phosphate dehydrogenase.
8. The vitamin required for transketolase reactions is: Thiamin.
9. The H^+ion acceptor of HMP shunt is: $NADP^+$.
10. Hormones enhancing the activity of the pathway are: Insulin and thyroid hormones.
11. Significance of HMP shunt:
    (*i*) Formation of NADPH which is required for various reductive biosynthetic reactions.
    (*ii*) Provides pentoses (xylulose,ribulose,ribose)for nucleotide and nucleic acid synthesis.
12. Reactions requiring NADPH are:
    (*i*) De Novo fatty acid synthesis
    (*ii*) Synthesis of cholesterol
    (*iii*) Synthesis of steroids
    (*iv*) Synthesis of Sphingolipids
    (*v*) Uronic acid pathway.
13. Disorders associated with (G–6–PD) glucose-6-phosphate dehydrogenase deficiency are: Haemolytic anemia and favism.
14. Wernicke–korsakoff syndrome is due to genetic defect in: Transketolase (thiamine deficiency).

Glycogen Metabolism

1. Storage form of glucose in animal body is: Glycogen.
2. Reasons for storage of glycogen:
    (*i*) It exerts no osmotic pressure
    (*ii*) It has a higher energy level than a corresponding weight of glucose.
3. Sites of glycogen storage: Liver and muscle.
4. Total amount of glycogen stored in skeletal muscle is greater than liver (though concentration of glycogen is higher in the liver) because: Skeletal muscle has greater mass as compared to liver.

5. The glycogen content of liver: 10 gm / 100 gm of tissue.
   The glycogen content of skeletal muscle: 1-2 gm / 100 ml.
6. Liver glycogen: Source of glucose for maintenance of blood glucose level.
   Muscle glycogen: source of energy
7. Rate limiting enzyme in glycogenesis is: Glycogen synthetase.
8. The protein on which a glycogen molecule is build is: Glycogenin.
9. Branching enzyme of glycogenesis is: Amylo – [1,4]' → [1,6] transglucosidase (Glycosyl-4, 6 transferase).
10. Stimulation of glycogenesis is by: Insulin, glucocorticoids, glucose.
11. Inhibition of glycogenesis is by: Increased concentration of glycogen, glucagon, epinephrine, norepinephrine
12. Rate limiting enzyme of glycogenolysis is: Phosphorylase.
13. Enzyme breaking ∝1 → 4 bonds in glycogenolysis is: Phosphorylase.
14. Enzyme breaking ∝1 → 6 bonds in glycogenolysis is: Amylo –1 → 6 glucosidase\Debranching enzyme.
15. Product of glycogenolysis in liver and muscle is: Glucose and glucose – 6 – PO_4 respectively.
16. In muscle final product of glycogenolysis is glucose – 6 – phosphate but not the glucose because it is deficient in: Glucose–6–phosphatase.
17. Stimulation of glycogenolysis is by: Epinephrine (liver, muscle), glucagon (liver)

Gluconeogenesis

1. Gluconeogenesis is: Synthesis of new glucose from noncarbohydrate precursors.
2. Sources of gluconeogenesis: Lactate , glucogenic amino acids, glycerol part of fat and propionyl CoA formed from odd chain fatty acids.
3. Major tissues involved in gluconeogenesis: Liver, kidney.
4. Key enzymes which regulate gluconeogenesis are: Pyruvate carboxylase, phosphoenol pyruvate carboxykinase, fructose-1, 6-bisphosphatase, and glucose 6 phosphatase, pyru vate carboxylase: Acetyl CoA activates the enzyme
   Fructose–1, 6– bisphosphatase: Inhibited by AMP and activated by ATP and citrate.
5. Hormonal regulation-Glucagon, epinephrine and glucocorticoids stimulate gluconeogenesis and insulin inhibits the process.
6. Glycerol is metabolized to: Pyruvate and dihydroxy acetone phosphate both of which can be converted to glucose in liver.
7. Propionic acid enters the main gluconeogenic pathway by being converted to: Succinyl CoA
8. Cori's cycle is concerned with: Transport of lactate from muscle and RBC's to liver and glucose formed from lactate back to muscle and RBC.
9. Amino acid not participating in gluconeogenesis is: Leucine.

Regulation of glycogen metabolism

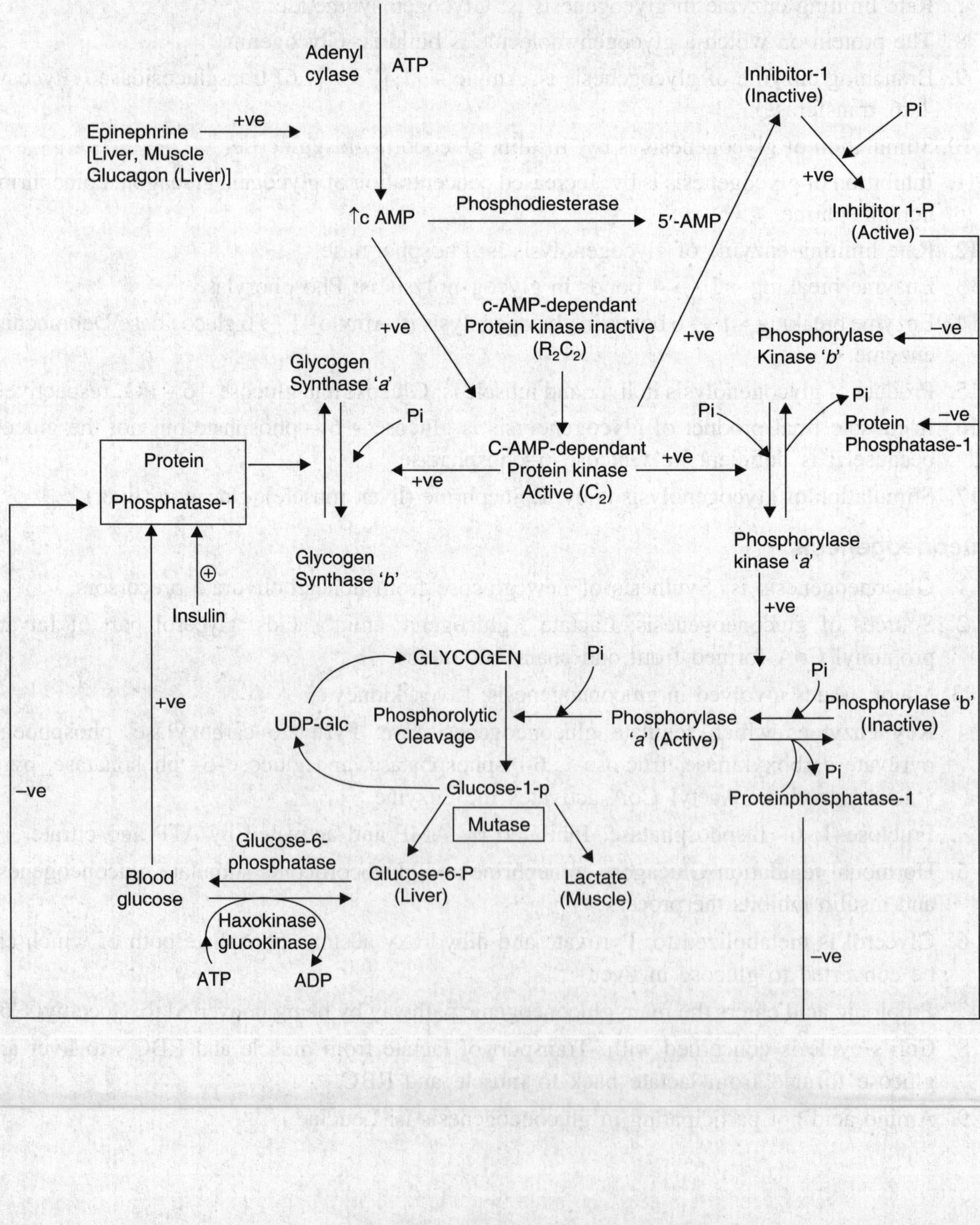

The cori cycle and glucose alanine cycle

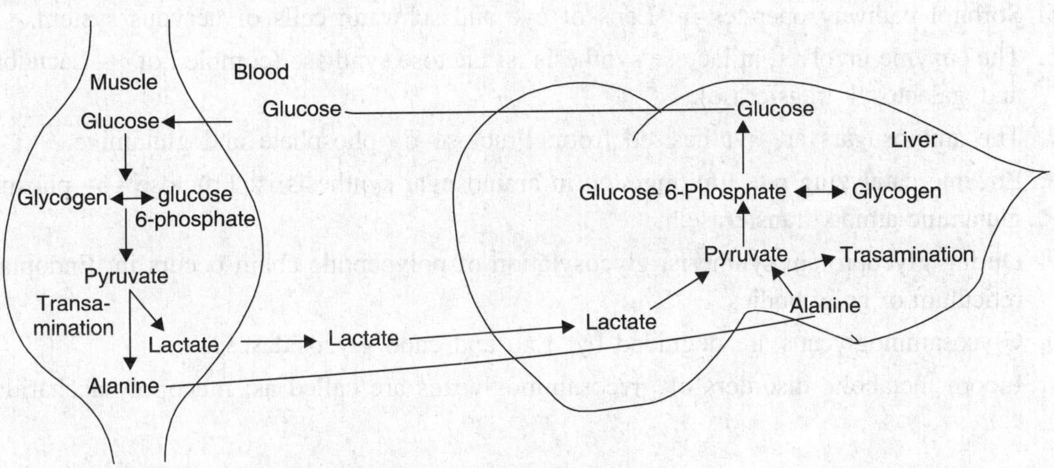

Other Pathways of Carbohydrate Metabolism

1. Glucose via uronic acid pathway forms: Glucuronic acid
2. Significance of the pathway is:
   (i) Source of UDP – Glucose which is used for glycogen formation
   (*ii*) Formation of glucuronosides for detoxifying the body
   (*iii*) Formation of ascorbic acid
   (*iv*) Formation of pentoses.
3. The carbon atom of glucose that is oxidized to form uronic acid: 6.
4. Uronic acid is incorporated into glycosaminoglycans as: UDP – Glucuronic acid.
5. Disorder associated with uronic acid pathway is: Essential pentosuria (L–Xylitol dehydrogenase deficiency).
6. Fructose is the major energy source for: Spermatozoa.
7. Excessive dietary fructose is harmful: Leads to increased synthesis of TG.
8. Fructose is more rapidly utilized because: Glucokinase and phosphofructokinase reactions are not encountered in fructose metabolism.
9. The enzyme cleaving fructose-1-phosphate is: Aldolase B or fructose-1- phosphate aldolase.
10. Disorders associated with fructose metabolism are:
    (*i*) Essential fructosuria (Fructokinase deficiency)
    (*ii*) Hereditary fructose intolerance (Aldolase B/Phosphofructoaldolase deficiency)
11. Galactose is required for synthesis of: Lactose, glycolipids, glycosaminoglycans and proteoglycans.
12. Most of galactose is converted to: Glucose.
13. Galactosemia is due to: Galactose -1- phosphate uridyl transferase deficiency (classical type), sometimes galactokinase deficiency (minor type).

14. Cataract formed in galactosemia is due to: Dulcitol (Galactitol).
15. Sorbitol pathway operates in: Lens of eye and schwann cells of nervous system.
16. The enzyme involved in lactose synthesis is: Lactose synthase (complex of ∝- Lactalbumin and galactosyl transferase).
17. The aminosugars are synthesised from: Fructose–6– phosphate and glutamine.
18. Enzyme catalyzing rate limiting step in aminosugar synthesis is: Fructose –6– phosphate-glutamine-amido transferase.
19. During glycoprotein synthesis, glycosylation of polypeptide chain occurs in: Endoplasmic reticulum or golgi bodies.
20. Glycosaminoglycans are degraded by: Exo and endo glycosidases.
21. Inborn metabolic disorders of glycosaminoglycans are called as: mucopolysaccharidoses.

SOLVED QUESTIONS

Q.1. Hydroxyethyl starch is a: **(AIPGME 1994)**

1. Vasodilator

2. Inotrope

3. Plasma expander

4. Diuretic.

Ans. 3

Hydroxyethyl starch is a plasma expander: There are some other plasma expanders-human albumin, dextran, degraded gelatin polymer, polyvinyl pyrrolidone.

Q.2. Which of the followoing is true regarding hydroxyl ethyl starch: **(AIPGME 2002)**

1. It is an anesthetic agent

2. It is a plasma expander

3. It is a crystalloid

4. Used as a nutritional agent.

Ans. 2

Hydroxyethyl starch, dextran, human albumin, degraded gelatin polymer, polyvinyl pyrrolidone are the examples of plasma expanders.

Q.3. Colonic bacteria on digestion of dietary fibres would give: **(AIIMS 2001)**

1. Free radicals

2. Glycerol

3. **Butyrate**
4. **Sucrose.**

Ans. 3

In herbivorous animals, such as ruminants dietary fiber includes mainly cellulose. Celluose is a major source of energy after it has been digested and converted by colonic microorganisms to small chain fatty acids (acetate, propionate and butyrate). These are then absorbed into the portal vein.Colonic fermentation may also contribute to human energy requirements.

Q.4. False about hereditary fructose intolerance is: **(AIIMS June 1998)**

1. **Deficiency of fructose 1-phosphate aldolase**
2. **Accumulation of fructose 1-phosphate in tissue**
3. **Hyperglycemia**
4. **Liver and kidneys are involved.**

Ans. 3

Hereditary fructose intolerance is because of deficiency of enzyme fructose -1- phosphate aldolase or aldolase B. Hence fructose-1- phosphate cannot be metabolized. Accumulation of fructose-1-phosphate will inhibit glycogen phosphorylase. This leads to accumulation of glycogen in liver. Glycogen metabolism in kidney is also affected. As glycogen is not degraded, it results into associated hypoglycemia.

Q.5. Viscocity of synovial fluid depends upon: **(AIIMS May 2002)**

1. **N-acetyl galactosamine**
2. **N-acetyl glucosamine**
3. **Glucuronic acid**
4. **Hyaluronic acid.**

Ans. 4

The viscocity and the plasticity of synovial fluid is because of presence of hyaluronic acid. Hyaluronic acid is a glycosaminoglycan and is composed of repeating disaccharide units of glucuronic acid and N-acetyl glucosamine.

Q.6. Oxaloacetate + Acetyl co A $\rightarrow$ Citrate + CoASH. This reaction is: **(AIIMS June 2000)**

1. **Reversible**
2. **Irreversible**
3. **Can be reversed by catalase**
4. **Competitive.**

Ans. 2

This is the first step of citric acid cycle. Oxaloacetate is condensed with acetyl CoA to form citrate. It is an irreversible reaction. This step is catalysed by the enzyme citrate synthase.

Q.7. Starvation and diabetes mellitus can lead on to ketoacidosis which of the following features is in favour of ketoacidosis due to diabetes mellitus.(AIIMS May 2001)

1. **Increase in glucagon/insulin, ratio, increased cAMP and increased blood glucose.**
2. **Decreased insulin, increased free fatty acid which is equivalent to blood glucose.**
3. **Decreased insulin, increased free fatty acids which is not equivalent to blood glucose.**
4. **Elevated insulin and free fatty acid, equivalent to blood glucose.**

Ans. **1**

In diabetes mellitus and starvation there is an increase in glucagon/ insulin ratio because of decreased insulin level and excess of glucagon. Glucagon acts by increasing cAMP level while insulin-inhibits cAMP production. As there is insulin deficiency, insulin dependent enzymes are less active. High glucagon level decreases the hepatic fructose-2,6-bisphosphate level, there by decreasing the utilization of glucose. All this effect leads to hyperglycemia.

Q.8. A child present with hepatomegaly and bilateral lenticular opacities. Deficiency of which of the following enzyme will not cause such features: (AIIMS Nov 2001)

1. **Galactose -1- phosphate uridyl transferase**
2. **UDP– galactose – 4 - epimerase**
3. **Galactokinase**
4. **Lactase.**

Ans. **4**

These symptoms are associated with galactosemia which results from the defect in galactose metabolism. Galactose-1-phosphate uridyl transferase, UDP-galactose-4-epimerase and galactokinase, all these enzymes are related with galactose utilization. Deficiency of any of the enzyme causes galactosemia.

Galactose-1-phosphate uridyl transferase deficiency: classical types.

Galactokinase deficiency: Minor type,

Epimerase deficiency: Rare types.

Lactase deficiency will not cause galactosemia as lactase is used to hydrolyse lactose into glucose and galactose. But lactase deficiency will cause deficiency of galactose.

Q.9. During Gluconeogenesis reducing equivalents from mitochondria to cytosol are transported by (AIIMS Nov 2002)

1. **Malate**
2. **Aspartate**
3. **Glutamate**
4. **Oxaloacetate.**

Ans. 1

In Gluconeogenesis, carboxylation of pyruvate to oxaloacetate occurs in mitochondria while the rest of the reactions are taking place in cytosol. Hence oxaloacetate has to be transported from mitochondria to cytosol.This is achieved by malate shuttle. Oxaloacetate is reduced by NADH+H$^+$ to malate. This malate is transported to the cytosol where it is reoxidised to oxaloacetate. In this reaction NADH+H$^+$ is regenerated. Thus reducing equivalents are transported to cytosol form mitochondria. Along with reducing equivalents oxaloacetate is transported to cytosol where further reactions of gluconeogenesis occurs.

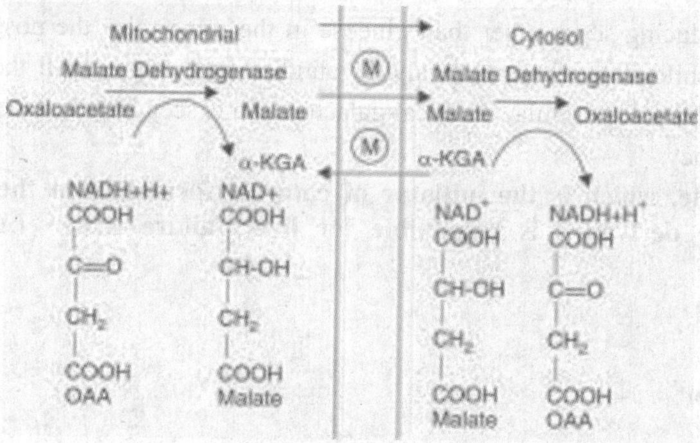

Q.10. The cause of hyperuricemia and gout in glucose–6–phosphatase deficiency is: (AIIMS Nov 2001)

1. **More formation of pentose**
2. **Decreased availability of glucose to tissue**
3. **Increased accumulation of sorbitol**
4. **Impaired degradation of free radicals**

Ans: 1

In Von Gierke's disease i.e. glucose-6-phosphatase deficiency hyperuricemia and gout is observed. Glucose-6-phosphatase converts glucose-6-phosphate into glucose. But its deficiency leads to accmulation of glucose-6-phosphate & hypoglycemia. This accumulated glucose-6-phosphate enters the HMP shunt & leads to increased production of pentoses. These pentoses are the substrates for phosphoribosyl pyrophosphate synthetase & result in increased production of purines.Thus purine turnover rate is increased causing its increased catabolism to uric acid resulting into hyperuricemia. Renal excretion of uric acid is decreased.

Q.11 A newborn infant refuses breast milk since the 2nd day of birth, vomits on force-feeding but accept glucose-water, develops diarrhea on the third day, by 5th day she is jaundiced with liver enlargements & eyes show signs of cataract, urinary

reducing sugar was positive but blood glucose estimated by glucose oxidation method was found low. The most likely cause is deficiency of: **(AIIMS May 2003)**

1. **Galactose-1-phosphate uridyl transferase**
2. **Beta galactosidase**
3. **Glucose-6- phosphatase**
4. **Galactokinase.**

Ans. 1

High levels of a reducing sugar other than glucose in the urine raise the possibility of galactose in urine. Also the child shows hepatomegaly & jaundice and cataract. All these are the signs & symptoms of classical galactosemia. Classical galactosemia is seen in galactose-1-phosphate uridyl transferase deficiency.

Q.12. The molecule, which is the initiator of cataract formation in the eyelens & whose 1-phosphate derivative is responible for liver failure is: **(AIIMS May 2005)**

1. **Sorbitol**
2. **Mannitol**
3. **Inositol**
4. **Galactitol**

Ans. 4

Galactitol or dulcitol is produced by reduction of free galactose. Galactose-1-phosphate uridyl transferase deficiency causes accumulation of galactose-1-phosphate in liver. This reduces bilirubin uptake and its conjugation by liver cells, increasing unconjugated bilirubin in blood. There is enlargement of liver and jaundice. Accumulated galactose-1- phosphate inhibits galactokinase so free galactose accumulates. Some of free galactose is reduced to galactitol or dulcitol. The accumulation of dulcitol in the lens results in cataract due to its osmotic effect.

Q.13. Fluoride inhibits which enzyme: **(AIPGME 1995)**

1. **Pyruvate kinase**
2. **Succinyl dehydrogenase**
3. **Enolase**
4. **Aldolase.**

Ans. 3

OR

Fluoride, used in the collection of blood samples for glucose estimations, inhibits the enzyme: **(AIPGME 2005)**

1. **Glucokinase**
2. **Hexokinase**

3. **Enolase**
4. **Glucose-6- phosphatase.**

Ans. 3

Fluoride inhibits the enzyme enolase. Sodium fluoride is used along with K-oxalate for collection of blood for blood glucose estimation. It inhibits in vitro glycolysis by inhibiting enzyme enolase. As glycolysis is prevented blood sugar is not utilized so it can be measured accurately.

Q.14. Metabolites in HMP shunt are all except: **(AIPGME 1995)**

1. **Glycerol-3-phosphate**
2. **Sedoheptulose-7-phosphate**
3. **Glyceraldehyde-3-phosphate**
4. **Xylulose-5-phosphate.**

Ans. 1

During HMP shunt xylulose-5- phosphate, sedoheptulose-7- phosphate and glyceraldehyde-3- phosphate are produced as intermediates of isomerization and transketolation reactions.

$$\text{Ribulose-5-phosphate} \xrightarrow{\text{Epimerase}} \text{Xylulose-5-phosphate.}$$

$$\text{Xylulose-5-phosphate + Ribose-5-phosphate} \xrightarrow{\text{Transketolase}} \text{Transketolase}$$

$$\text{Sedoheptulose-7-phosphate + Glylceraldehyde-3-phosphate}$$

While glycerol-3-phosphate is produced during gluconeogenesis form glycerol.

Q.15. Malate shuttle is seen to occur in: **(AIPGME 1998)**

1. **Glycolysis**
2. **Glycogenolysis**
3. **HMP Shunt**
4. **Gluconeogenesis.**

Ans. 4

Explanation same as given in Q. 9

Q.16. Glucose may be synthesised from: **(AIIMS Nov 2002)**

1. **Glycerol**
2. **Adenine**
3. **Guanine**
4. **Palmitic acid.**

Ans. 1

Adenine and guanine are nitrogen bases (purines) They are required for nucleotide and nucleic acid synthesis. Palmitic acid can not be used for glucose synthesis because acetyl CoA can not be reconverted back to pyruvate. Even chain fatty acids are not substrates for gluconeogenesis.

Glycerol can be converted to glycerol-3-phosphate which is then oxidized to dihydroxy acetone phosphate, an intermediate of glycolysis or gluconeogenesis.

Q.17. Enzyme to both common in gluconeogenesis and glycolysis pathway is:

(AIPGME 1997)

1. **Phosphofructokinase**
2. **Fructose 2, 6 - bisphosphatase**
3. **Hexokinase**
4. **Glucose-6-phosphatase.**

Ans. **2**

Phosphofructokinase, hexokinase and pyruvate kinase catalyse irreversible steps in glycolysis. Fructose 1,6-bisphosphatase, glucose-6- phosphatase, pyruvate carboxylase and phosphoenol pyruvate carboxykinase are corresponding key gluconeogenic enzymes. Fructose 2,6,-bisphosphatase is an enzyme of Rapaport Leubering cycle (BPG shunt). In erythrocytes this pathway is operative. 2,3-BPG is produced from fructose-6-phosphate.Then fructose 2,6 bisphosphatase hydrolyses fructose-2,6 bisphosphate into 3-phosphoglycerate.

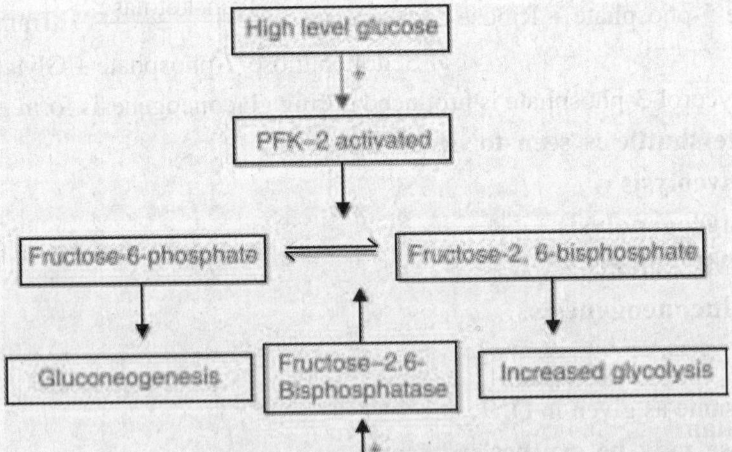

Q.18. The major fate of glucose-6-phosphate in tissue in a well fed state is:

(AIPGME 1997)

1. **Hydrolysis to glucose**
2. **Conversion to glycogen**
3. **Isomerization to fructose-6-phosphate**
4. **Conversion to ribulose-5-phosphate.**

Ans. 2

In a well fed state glucose-6-phosphate is converted to glycogen.. Glycogen is the storage form of carbohydrates in the human body. Its major function is to provide a source of glucose for maintenance of blood glucose level.

Q.19. Gluconeogenesis occurs in all except: (AIPGME 1996)

1. **Glycerol**
2. **Amino acid**
3. **Lactic acid**
4. **Palmitate.**

Ans. 4

Even chain fatty acids can not be converted to glucose. Oxidation of even chain fatty acids gives acetyl CoA and conversion of pyruvate to acetyl CoA irreversible reaction. There is no any enzyme that converts acetyl CoA to pyruvate. But propionyl CoA formed from odd chain fatty acids is one of the substrate of gluconeogenesis along with glycerol, amino acids and lactic acid.

Q.20. Glucose can be synthesized from all of the following except: (AIPGME 1997)

1. **Acetoacetate**
2. **Lactic acid**
3. **Glycerol**
4. **Amino acid.**

Ans. 1

Acetoacetate is a ketone body. During ketolysis, it is activated to acetoacetyl CoA which gives acetyl CoA. Acetyl CoA can not be reconverted back to pyruvate so acetoacetate can not be utilized for gluconeogenesis.

Q.21. Pyruvate can be converted directly into all the following except: (AIPGME 2000)

1. **Phosphoenol pyruvate**
2. **Alanine**
3. **Acetyl CoA**
4. **Lactate.**

Ans. 1

Conversion of phosphoenol pyruvate to pyruvate is irreversible reaction so pyruvate can not be directly converted to phosphoenol pyruvate.First in the mitochondria pyruvate is converted to oxaloacetate which is reduced to malate. Then malate is transported to cytosol where it is reconverted back to oxaloacetate which is then converted by phosphoenol pyruvate.

Pyruvate undergoes transamination to form alanine. Pyruvate undergoes oxidative decarboxylation to acetyl coA. Pyruvate is reduced to lactate.

Q.22. The rate limiting enzyme in glycolysis is: (AIPGME 2000)

1. **Phosphofructokinase**
2. **Glucose-6-dehydrogenase**
3. **Glucokinase**
4. **Pyruvate kinase.**

Ans. 1

Phosphofructokinase is the rate limiting enzyme and the major regulatory enzyme of glycolysis. AMP and fructose-2,6-bisphosphate are its activators while ATP and citrate are inhibitors.

Glucokinase and pyruvate kinase are also regulatory enzymes of glycolysis. Glucose-6- phosphate dehydrogenase is the rate limiting enzyme in HMP shunt.

Q.23. An enzyme involved in the catabolism of fructose to pyruvate in the liver is: (AIPGME 2003)

1. **Glyceraldehyde-3-phosphate dehydrogenase**
2. **Phosphoglucomutase**
3. **Lactate dehydrogenase**
4. **Glucokinase.**

Ans. 1

Fructose is phosphorylated to fructose-1-phosphate by fructokinase. Fructose-1-phosphate is then cleaved by the enzyme fructose-1-phosphate aldolase or aldolase B to glyceraldehyde and dihydroxyacetone phosphate. The glyceraldehyde is phosphorylated to glyceraldehyde-3-phosphate which is acted upon by glyceraldehyde-3-phosphate dehydrogenase. It then enters into glycolytic pathway to form pyruvate, Lactate dehydrogenase is required for interconversion between pyruvate and lactate. Glucokinase is specific for glucose only.

Q.24. A Young man finds that every time he eats dairy products he feels very uncomfortable. His stomach becomes distended. He develops gas and diarrhoea frequently. These symptoms do not appear when he eats foods other than dairy products. Which of the following is most likely enzyme in which this young man is deficient? (AIPGME 2004)

1. **α-amylase**
2. **β-galactosidase**
3. **α-glucosidase**
4. **Sucrase.**

Ans. 2

β-Galactosidase hydrolyses lactose to galactose and glucose. Deficiency of this enzyme causes inability to utilise lactose. Lactose accumulates in the gut where it is acted upon by bacteria to produce organic acids. These take up water into bowels by osmotic effect. Irritant diarrhoea is thus produced.

Q.25. Substrate level phosphorylation is seen in the conversion of: (AIPGME 2002)

1. **Acetoacetate to α-ketoglutarate**
2. **Succinyl CoA to succinate**
3. **Fumarate to malate**
4. **Succinate to fumarate.**

Ans. 2

In the conversion of succinyl CoA to succinate a high energy phosphate is generated from the energy trapped in the thioester bond of succinyl CoA. The enzyme is succinate thiokinase. A molecule of GDP is phosphorylated to GTP. The GTP can be converted to ATP by reacting with an ADP molecule. Thus without entering into electron transport chain at substrate level only ATP is generated.

Q.26. A genetic disorder renders fructose 1,6-bisphosphatase in liver less sensitive to regulation by fructose 2,6-bisphosphate. All of the following metabolic changes are observed in this disorder except: (AIPGME 2004)

1. **Level of fructose 1,6- bisphosphate is higher than normal**
2. **Level of fructose 1,6- bisphosphate is lower than normal**
3. **Less pyruvate is formed**
4. **Less ATP is generated.**

Ans. 2

Fructose 2,6-bisphosphate is an inhibitor of fructose 1,6-bisphosphatase. If because of genetic disorder the sensitivity of this enzyme to fructose 2,6-bisphosphate is lost then the enzyme is not inhibited , so there is more and more conversion of fructose 1,6-bisphosphate into fructose-6-phosphate by the enzyme fructose 1,6-bisphosphatase.

Q.27. Substrate level phosphorylation is catalysed by: (AIIMS June 1998)

1. **Succinate dehydrogenase**
2. **Thiokinase**
3. **Malate dehydrogenase**
4. **Hexokinase.**

Ans. 2

Explanation same as Q.25

Q.28. Enzymes concerned with the citric acid cycle are found in the

1. **Nucleus**
2. **Ribosomes**
3. **Mitochondria**
4. **Non particulate system.**

Ans. 3

All the enzyme of citric acid cycle are located inside the mitochondria.

Q.29. Substrate level phosphorylation occurs during:

1. **Isocitrate ⟶ Oxalosuccinate**
2. **α-KGA ⟶ Succinyl CoA**
3. **Succinyl CoA ⟶ Succinate**
4. **Succinate ⟶ Fumarate.**

Ans. 3

In the conversion of succinyl CoA to succinate a high energy phosphate is generated from the energy trapped in the thioester bond of succinyl CoA. The enzyme is succinate thiokinase. A molecule of GDP is phosphorylated to GTP. The GTP can be converted to ATP by reacting with an ADP molecule. During conversion of isocitrate to oxalosuccinate, and ∝- ketoglutarate to succinyl CoA and NADH is generated while in the conversion of succinate to fumarate $FADH_2$ is generated . Both NADH and $FADH_2$ enters in electron transport chain for ATP synthesis .

Q.30. The dental plaque is formed by the enzymatic reactions of which of the following:

1. **Glucose and lipid**
2. **Sucrose and protein**
3. **Glucose and saliva**
4. **Sucrose and saliva.**

Ans. 4

Q.31. Which of the following is a multienzyme complex:

1. **Glucose-6-phosphate dehydrogenase**
2. **Lactate dehydrogenase**
3. **α-ketoglutarate dehydrogenase**
4. **Isocitrate dehydrogenase.**

Ans. 3

The enzyme α-ketoglutarate dehydrogenase is a multienzyme complex having 3 enzyme proteins and 5 coenzymes.

Q.32. The key enzyme for gluconeogenesis is:

1. **Pyruvate carboxylase**
2. **Fructose 1,6-bisphophatase**
3. **Glucose-6-phosphatase**
4. **Phosphoenol pyruvate carboxykinase.**

Ans. 1

Pyuvate carboxylase is a rate limiting enzyme of gluconeogenesis it catalyzes the conversion of pyruvate to oxaloacetic acid.

Q.33. The enzyme involved in the first committed step of glycolysis is:

1. PFK

2. Glucose-6-phosphatase

3. Hexokinase

4. Enolase.

Ans. 3

The enzymes catalyzing committed steps (irreversible reactions) of glycolysis are:

(1) Hexokinase

(2) Phosphofructokinase

(3) Pyruvate kinase.

Q.34. NADPH is produced by:

1. Glycolysis

2. Citric acid cycle

3. Hexose monophosphate shunt

4. Glycogenesis.

Ans. 3

The major metabolic role of the hexose monophosphate shunt is to provide cytoplasmic NADPH for reductive biosynthesis of fatty acid, cholesterol and steroids.

Q.35. Increased concentration of cytosolic Ca promotes:

1. Glycogenesis

2. Glycogenolysis

3. Gluconeogenesis

4. Glycolysis.

Ans. 2

Ca binds with calmodulin (Ca binding protein) which activates glycogen phosphorylase promoting glycogenolysis

Q.36. What high energy phosphate compound is formed in the citric acid cycle through substrate level phosphorylation:

1. ATP

2. TTP

3. ITP

4. GTP

Ans. 4

Substrate level phosphorylation step is conversion of succinyl CoA to succinate.The energy trapped in the thioester bond of succinyl CoA is then stored in the form of GTP. The enzyme succinate thiokinase phosphorylate GDP to GTP.

Q.37. Which one of the following is the correct sequential order in which the given enzymes of Kreb's cycle are formed after a molecule of acetyl CoA:

1. **Citrate, Oxaloacetate, Ketoglutarate**
2. **Ketoglutarate, Oxaloacetate, Citrate**
3. **Citrate, Ketoglutarate, Oxaloacetate**
4. **Oxaloacetate, Ketoglutarate, Citrate.**

Ans. **3**

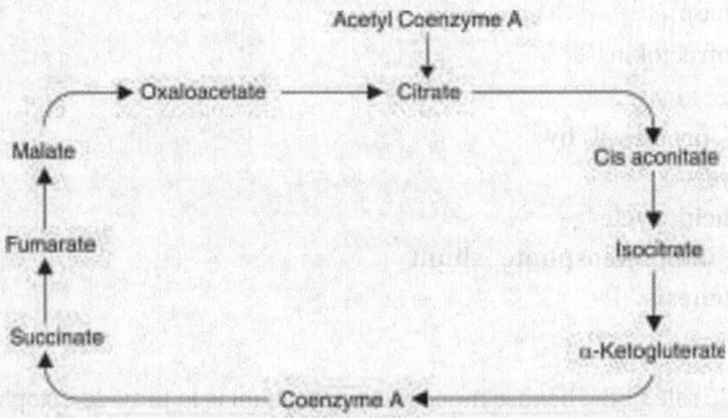

TCA Cycle

Q.38. The conversion of glucose-6-phosphate to fructose-6-phosphate is an example of which of the following reactions:

1. **Phosphate transfer**
2. **Isomerisation**
3. **Dehydration**
4. **Aldol cleavage.**

Ans. **2**

The conversion of glucose-6-phosphate to fructose-6-phosphate is an example of isomerization reactions catalysed by isomerase enzyme. These enzymes can produce optical, geometric or positional isomers of substrates.

Q.39. Production of fructose in seminal fluid is by following steps:

1. **Glucose-6-phosphate < fructose-6-phosphate < fructose**
2. **Glucose-6-phosphate < sorbitol phosphate < fructose phosphate < fructose**
3. **Glucose-6-phosphate < glucose < sorbitol < fructose**
4. **Glucose-6-Phosphate < fructose-1-phosphate < fructose.**

Ans. **3**

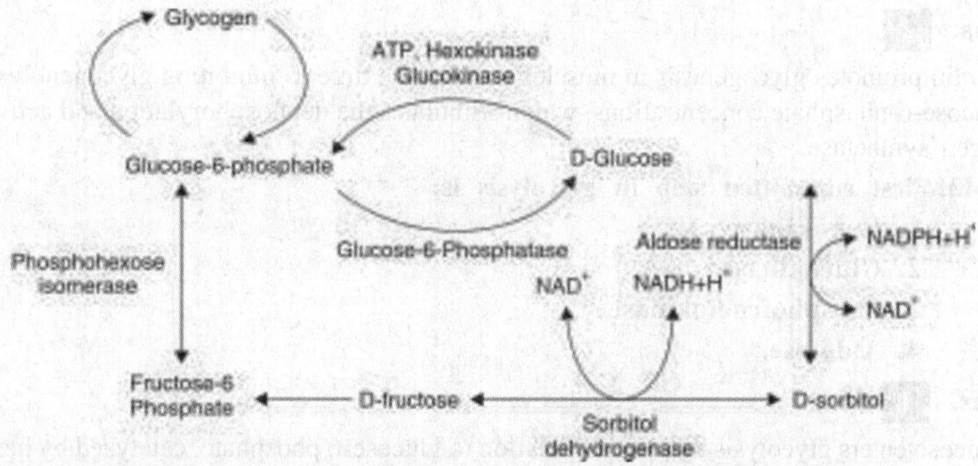

Q.40. Muscle cannot make use of glycogen for energy due to the absence of:

1. **Glucose-6-phosphatase**
2. **Glucokinase**
3. **Phosphorylase**
4. **Phosphoglucomutase:**

Ans. **3**

Muscles cannot make use of glycogen for energy as it contains phosphorylase which is a dimer, each monomer containing one molecule of PLP. The two forms of the enzyme are phosphorylase a, which is phosphorylated and active either in the presence or absence of 5' AMP, and phosphorylase b, which is dephosphorylated and active only in the presence of 5' AMP. During exercise the level of 5' AMP rises and provides fuel for the muscles.

Q.41. Skeletal muscle is deficient in:

1. **Glucose-6-phosphatase**
2. **Hexokinase**
3. **Isomerase**
4. **Phosphofructokinase**

Ans. **1**

The conversion of glucose-6-phosphate to glucose is catalyzed by glucose -6 phosphatase which is present in liver and kidney but absent in muscle and adipose tissue, which therefore, cannot export glucose into the blood stream.

Q.42. Glycogen synthetase is increased by:

1. **Cortisone**
2. **Insulin**

3. **GH**
4. **Epinephrine.**

Ans. 2

Insulin promotes glycogenesis in muscles at the same time as inhibiting glycogenolysis by raising glucose-6-phosphate concentrations, which stimulates the dephosphorylation and activation of glycogen synthetase.

Q.43. First committed step in glycolysis is:

1. **Hexokinase**
2. **Glucokinase**
3. **Phosphofructokinase**
4. **Aldolase.**

Ans. 1

Glucose enters glycolysis by phosphorylation to glucose-6 phosphate, catalyzed by hexokinase, using ATP as the phosphate donor.

Q.44. The rate of absorption of sugars by small intestine is highest for:

1. **Disaccharides**
2. **Polysaccharides**
3. **Hexoses**
4. **Pentose.**

Ans. 3

The increase in blood glucose after a test dose of a carbohydrate compared with that after an equivalent amount of glucose is known as the glycemic index. Glucose and galactose have an index of 1, as do lactose, maltose, isomaltose and trehalose, which give rise to these monosaccharides on hydrolysis. Fructose and the sugar alcohols are absorbed less rapidly and have a lower glycemic index as does sucrose.

Q.45. Which metabolite of TCA cycle is used in detoxification of ammonia in brain:

1. **Alpha ketogluterate**
2. **Ornithine**
3. **Oxaloacetate**
4. **Glycine.**

Ans. 4

Tha ammonia produced by tissue are rapidly removed from circulation by the liver and converted to urea. This is very essential as ammonia is toxic to CNS. Should portal blood bypass the liver, systemic blood ammonia level may rise to toxic levels. Ammonia may be toxic to the brain in part because it reacts with ∝-Ketogluterate to form glutamate. The resulting depleted levels of ∝-Ketogluterate then impaired function of TCA cycle in neurons.

Q.46. 1 molecule of glucose forms ____ molecules of pyruvate:

1. 1
2. 2
3. 3
4. 5.

Ans. **2**

During glycolysis, two molecules of triose phosphate are formed per molecule of glucose, two molecules of ATP are generated at this stage per molecule of glucose.

Q.47. Mc Ardles disease is due to the deficiency of:

1. Glucose - 1 - phosphatase
2. Glucose - 1, 6 - diphosphatase
3. Glucose - 6 - phosphatase
4. Myophosphorylase.

Ans. **4**

This disease is also characterized as myophosphorylase deficiency. During this muscles have abnormally high glycogen content (2.5 to 4.1%) and little or no lactate in blood after exercise.

Q.48. The main pathways of metabolism in brain are:

1. Glycolysis and citric acid cycle
2. Glycogenolysis and Gluconeogenesis
3. Embden-Meyerhof pathway and H.M.P shunt pathway
4. Glycogenolysis and citric acid cycle.

Ans. **1**

The brain can metabolize ketone bodies to meet about 20% of its energy requirements the remainder must be supplied by glucose.So there are two pathways that takes place in brain they are glycolysis and amino acid metabolism.

Q.49. Which of the following is not a product of HMP shunt:

1. NADPH
2. D fructose - 6 - phosphate
3. D sedoheptulose 7 phosphate
4. D glyceraldehyde - 3 - phosphate.

Ans. **1**

NADPH is not the product of the HMP shunt. It is co-enzyme which acts as a hydrogen acceptor at different steps.

Q.50. An essential for the conversion of glucose to glycogen in liver is:

1. UTP

2. GTP

3. Pyruvate kinase

4. Guanosine.

Ans. 1

UTP is essential for the conversion of glucose to glycogen. As glucose-1-phosphate reacts with GTP to form active nucleoside UDP- glucose and pyrophosphate. The glycogen synthase catalyzes the formation of a glycoside bond between C_1 of the activated glucose of UDP- glucose and C_4 of the terminal glucose residue of glycogen, liberating uridine diphosphate (UDP). A preexisting 'glycogen primer' must be present to initiate this reaction. This primer is formed on a primer known as glycogenin.

Q.51. All are true regarding glucose-6-phosphate deficiency except:

1. Hyperuricemia

2. Hyperglycemia

3. Defective cori cycle

4. Increased mobilization of glycogen from liver.

Ans. 2

The glucose-6-phosphate deficiency (von-Gierke's disease) shows the following characteristics-

(a) Liver cells and renal tubule cells loaded with glycogen.

(b) Hypoglycemia

(c) Lactic acidemia

(d) Ketosis

(e) Hyperlipemia

(f) Hyperuricemia.

Q.52. Kerb's cycle does not occur in:

1. Muscles

2. RBC's

3. Heart

4. All the above.

Ans. 2

Kreb's cycle does not takes place in RBCs. As they lack mitochondria and hence are wholly reliant on glycolysis and the pentose phosphate pathway.

Q.53. Aldose sugar is converted to ketose sugar by:

1. Aldolase

2. Isomerase

3. Decarboxylase

4. **Oxido-reductase.**

Ans. **2**

Aldose sugar is converted to ketose sugar by isomerase for eg. Fructose and glucose have same molecular formula. They differs only in the presence of keto group at position-2 (anomeric carbon) and aldehyde group at position-1 respectively

Q.54. Starch and glycogen are both polymers of:

1. **Mannose**
2. **alpha-glucose**
3. **Beta-glucose**
4. **Fructose.**

Ans. **2**

Starch is a homopolymer of glucose forming an ∝- glucosidic chain, called a glucosan or glucan. Where as the glycogen is the highly branched structure with chains of 12-14 α-D glucopyranose residues [in $\alpha(1 \rightarrow 4)$ glucosidic linkage] with branching by means of $\alpha\,(1 \rightarrow 6)$ glucosidic bonds.

Q.55. Which of the following is not a polymer of glucose:

1. **Glycogen**
2. **Cellulose**
3. **Amylose**
4. **Inulin.**

Ans. **4**

Inulin is the polymer of fructose.

Q.56. HMP shunt is of great importance in cellular metabolism because it produces:

1. **ATP**
2. **ADP**
3. **Acetyl CoA**
4. **NADPH.**

Ans. **4**

The HMP shunt is of great importance as it is active in liver, adipose tissue, adrenal cortex, thyroid, erythrocytes, testis and lactating mammary gland. Its activity is low in non lactating mammary gland and skeletal muscles. These tissues use NADPH as reductive synthases. As this is the characteristic product of the pentose phosphate pathway which is not produced in glycolysis.

Q.57. Inhibition of glycolysis by O_2 is known as:

1. **Muni effect**
2. **Pasteur effect**

3. **Hill reaction**
4. **Gluconeogenesis.**

Ans. 2

The inhibition of phosphofructokinase-1 by citrate and ATP is the explanation of the sparing action of fatty acid oxidation on glucose oxidation and also of the pasteur effect, whereby aerobic oxidation (via the citric acid cycle) inhibits the anaerobic degradation by glucose.

Q.58. Sites where HMP shunts can occur include:

1. **Liver**
2. **WBC**
3. **Lactating mammary gland**
4. **All.**

Ans. 4

Same as (57).

Q.59. By which of the following anticoagulants used in estimating blood glucose, Glycolysis is prevented: (AIIMS Nov 2005)

1. **EDTA.**
2. **Heparin.**
3. **Sodium fluoride.**
4. **Sodium citrate.**

Ans. 3

Sodium fluoride is used as an anticoagulant during blood glucose estimation as it inhibits the enzyme enolase required for the conversion of phoshoglycerate to phosphoenol pyruvate and so the Glycolysis is also inhibited. Due to this property of sodium fluoride this will helps in the correct determination of the blood glucose level as Glycolysis will not be able to affect the level of glucose.

Q.60. A PHC medical officer wants to send blood sample for glucose estimation to a district hospital. What is the preservative that should be used? (AIIMS Nov 2006)

1. **EDTA.**
2. **Calcium oxalate**
3. **Potassium oxalate + NaF.**
4. **Potassium oxalate + Nal**

Ans. 3

It is estimated that plasma glucose reduces by 10 mg% for each hour delay from the time of blood drawing because the RBCs in the sample are still alive and they extract glucose for Glycolysis giving the false low value of blood glucose. To avoid this sodium fluoride is added to inhibit Glycolysis as it inhibits enolase step of Glycolysis. Potassium oxalate sequestrates calcium ions hence used as anticoagulants.

Q.61. Mucopolysaccharide hyaluronic acid is present in: (AIPGEE 2007)

1. **Vitreous humour.**
2. **Cornea.**
3. **Blood vessels.**
4. **Synovial fluid.**

Ans. 1

Hyaluronic acid consists of an unbranched chain of repeating disaccharide units containing Glc UA and Glc Nac. Hyaluronic acid is present in bacteria and is widely distributed among various animals and tissues, including synovial fluid, the vitreous body of the eye, cartilage and loose connective tissues.

Q.62. HMP shunt occurs in: (AIPGEE 2007)

1. **Cytosol.**
2. **Mitochondria.**
3. **Endoplasmic reticulum.**
4. **Golgi apparatus.**

Ans. 1

The enzymes of HMP shunt are located in the cytosol. The tissues such as, liver, adipose tissue, adrenal gland, erythrocytes, testis and lactating mammary gland, are highly active in HMP shunt. The pathway starts with glucose-6-phosphate. As such, no ATP is directly utilized or produced in HMP pathway.

Q.63. In HMP shunt oxidative phase generates: (AIPGEE 2007)

1. **Ribose.**
2. **NADPH.**
3. **Pyruvate.**
4. **Lactate**

Ans. 2

HMP shunt oxidase phase generates NADPH. Glucose-6- phosphate dehydrogenase is an NADP dependent enzyme that converts glucose-6 –phosphate to 6-phosphogluconolactone. The latter is then hydrolyzed by the gluconolactone hydrolase to 6- phosphogluconate. The next reaction involving the synthesis of NADPH is catalyzed by 6-phosphogluconate dehydrogenase to produce 3-keto-6 phosphogluconate, which then undergoes decarboxylation to give ribulose –5-phosphate.

NOTES

3

Lipids

1. Lipids are:
   (a) Heterogeneous group of compounds:
   (b) Related by their physical rather than by their chemical properties
   (c) Esters of fatty acids with different alcohols.
2. The common physical property of lipids is:
   (a) Insoluble in water
   (b) Soluble in nonpolar solvents like ether, chloroform etc.
3. Lipids are compounds of mainly: C, H and O. Sometime carry-P, N and S also.
4. In lipids: The ratio of H and O is generally much higher than in H_2O and carbohydrates.
5. Simple lipids are– Esters of fatty acids with various alcohols.
6. Types of simple lipids are:
   (a) Triacylglycerol or neutral fat
   (b) Waxes
7. In fats the alcohol is: Glycerol.
   In waxes the alcohol is: Higher monohydric aliphatic alcohols.
8. Complex lipids are: Fatty acids esterified with alcohols but in addition they contain other groups.
9. Examples of complex lipids are:
   (a) Phospholipids - Fatty acid + Alcohol + phosphoric acid + N_2 – base
   (b) Glycolipids - Fatty acid + Sphingosine + carbohydrate
   (c) Lipoproteins - Lipid-protein complexes
   (d) Sulfolipids - Lipids characterised by possessing sulphate.
10. Two types of phospholipids are:
    (a) Phosphoglycerides (glycerol as an alcohol)
    (b) Sphingomyelins (Sphingosine as alcohol).

11. Derived lipids are: Derived from simple or compounds lipids by their hydrolysis.
12. Fatty acids, glycerol and steroids are called: Derived lipids.
13. Fatty acids are: Aliphatic carboxylic acids (R-COOH) where COOH represents the functional group.
14. In naturally occurring unsaturated fatty acids, the double bonds are in: Cis configuration.
15. The essential fatty acids include: Linoleic acid, linolenic acid and arachidonic acid.
16. ω_3–Family lipids: Timnodonic and linolenic acids
    ω_6–Family lipids: Linoleic and arachidonic acids
    ω_9–Family lipids: Oleic acid.
17. Precursor of eicosanoids is: Arachidonic acid.
18. Eicosanoids are: Prostaglandins, thromboxanes, leukotrienes and lipoxins
19. Common feature of all prostaglandins:
    (a) Cyclopentane ring
    (b) –OH group at 15th position
    (c) Trans double bond at 13th position.
20. Thromboxanes have: Cyclopentane ring interrupted with an oxygen atom.
21. Leukotrienes have: No ring in its structure and have 3 conjugated double bonds.
22. Different phospholipids present are: Phosphatidyl choline (lecithin), phosphatidyl ethanolamine (cephalin), phosphatidyl serine, phosphatidyl inositol (lipositol), cardiolipin.
23. Examples of sphingolipids- Sphingophospholipid (sphingomyelin), glycolipid.
24. Deficiency of dipalmitoyl lecithin (surfactant) leads to: Neonatal respiratory distress syndrome.
25. Sphingomyelins consist of: Ceramide + phosphoric acid + choline.
26. Ceramide is formed from: Sphingosine and fatty acid.
27. A glycolipid found in erythrocyte membrane is: Lactosyl ceramide.
28. Fetal lung maturity can be evaluated by: Lecithin to sphingomyelin ratios.
29. Types of gangliosides: GM_1, GM_2, GM_3.
30. Simples ganglioside is: GM_3.
31. Gangliosides are composed of: Sphingosine, a long chain fatty acid, sialic acid, glucose and galactose.
32. Steroids contain: Cyclopentanoperhydro- phenanthrene nucleus.
33. Structure of cholesterol:
    (a) 27 carbon atoms
    (b) Cyclopentanoperhydro phenanthrene ring
    (c) – OH group at C_3
    (d) Double bond between C_5 and C_6.
34. Cholesterol estimation is commonly done by: Zak's reaction.

35. Examples of amphipathic lipids are: Fatty acids, phospholipids, bile salts and cholesterol.
36. Examples of hydrophobic lipids are:Triacylglycerol and cholesteryl ester.
37. Plant sterol is: Ergosterol.
38. Principal sterol excreted in faeces: Coprosterol.
39. Association of lipids with proteins for transport in plasma is called: Lipoproteins.
40. Dietary TG is transported in plasma by: Chylomicrons.
41. Chylomicrons is synthesized in: Intestine.
42. Endogenous TG is transported in plasma by: VLDL.
43. Predominant lipid in LDL is: Cholesterol.
44. The apolipoprotein of LDL is: Apo B_{100}.
45. Longest single polypeptide chain is found in: Apo B_{100}.
46. LDL: Transport cholesterol from liver to tissues.
47. HDL: Transport cholesterol to liver.
48. Predominant lipid in HDL is: Phospholipid.

Metabolism of Fatty Acids

1. Site of fatty acid synthesis is: Liver, adipose tissue, brain, kidney and mammary glands.
2. Location of the pathway is: Cytoplasm.
3. The starting material for de novo synthesis of fatty acids is: Acetyl CoA.
4. Donor for the 2 carbon fragments during fatty acid synthesis is: Malonyl CoA.
5. CO_2 required for malonyl CoA production is provided by: Bicarbonate (HCO_3)
6. Rate limiting step in fatty acid synthesis is: Conversion of acetyl CoA to malonyl CoA by enzyme acetyl CoA carboxylase.
7. The enzymes responsible for fatty acid synthesis are present in a single polypeptide chain and are called as: Fatty acid synthase complex.
8. Fatty acid synthase complex occurs as: Homodimer.
9. Each monomeric unit contains: 6 enzymes and an ACP molecule (Total 7 in each monomer) Homo dimer has: 7 x 2 = 14 enzymes.
10. Coenzymes and cofactors required are: Biotin , NADPH, Mn^{++}.
11. Activators of acetyl CoA carboxylase are:- Citrate

Insulin inhibitors: Palmitoyl CoA and glucagon.

12. For synthesis of one molecule of palmitate (16 carbon) the cycle needs: 7 turns.
13. Net reaction: 8 Acetyl CoA + 7 ATP + 14 NADPH + $14H^+$ + $H_2O \rightarrow$ Palmitate + 7 ADP + 7 Pi + 8 CoA- SH + 14 $NADP^+$.
14. Two types of elongation systems–
    Endoplasmic reticulum system
    Mitochondrial elongation system.
15. Reducing equivalents for the pathway are provided by: Pentose Phosphate Pathway.

16. Fatty acid oxidation occurs in: Mitochondrial matrix.
17. End products of fatty acid oxidation are: NADH, $FADH_2$, Acetyl CoA.
18. Carrier for transport of long chain fatty acids through mitochondrial membrane is: Carnitine.
19. Carnitine (β–hydroxy-trimethylammonium butyrate) is synthesised from amino acid: Lysine, methionine.
20. Net reaction is:
    Palmitoyl CoA + 7 FAD + 7 NAD^+ + 7 H_2O + 7CoASH → 8 Acetyl CoA + 7$FADH_2$ + 7 NADH + 7 H^+.
21. Net ATP formed from β oxidation and TCA oxidation of one molecule of palmitate: 129 (131- 2).
22. Palmitic acid needs: 7 cycles of β oxidation which give 8 acetyl CoA molecules.
23. β Oxidation of odd chain fatty acids produces: Propionyl CoA at the last step.
24. Fate of propionyl CoA: Enters Gluconeogenesis
25. Long chain fatty acids are oxidised by: α–oxidation.
26. Carbon atoms removed during each turn of α–oxidation is: Single carbon atom.
27. α-Oxidation pathway do not need: Initial activation of FA.
28. Disease associated with α–oxidation pathway: Refsum's disease.
29. α–oxidation of fatty acids occur in: Brain.
30. ATP synthesised during α-oxidation of fatty acids: Nil.
31. Unsaturated fatty acids are oxidised by: Modified β-oxidation.
32. ω–oxidation of fatty acids produces: Dicarboxyllic acids.
33. β–oxidation of very long chain fatty acids takes place in: Peroxisomes.
34. β–oxidation in peroxisomes forms: H_2O_2 which is detoxified by catalase.
35. End products of β–oxidation in peroxisomes is: Octanoyl CoA + acetyl CoA.
36. Inherited absence of peroxisomes in all tissues produces: Zellweger's syndrome.
37. Primary ketone body is: Acetoacetate.
38. Secondary ketone bodies are: Beta hydroxy butyrate and acetone.
39. Site of ketone body synthesis is: Liver mitochondria.
40. Substrate for formation of ketone bodies: Acetyl CoA obtained from oxidation of free fatty acids.
41. Enzyme involved in the synthesis of ketone bodies is: Mitochondrial HMG CoA synthase
42. Cleavage of HMG CoA yields: Acetoacetate and acetyl CoA.
43. Concentration of total ketone bodies in the blood of well fed individuals is: Less than 1 mg/100 ml.
44. Daily loss of ketone bodies via urine is: less than 1 mg/24 hrs.
45. The predominant ketone body present in blood and urine in ketosis: Beta hydroxy butyrate
46. Oxidation of ketone body yields: 2 molecules of acetyl CoA.

47. Energy yield from oxidation of acetoacetate is: 23 ATP.
48. Energy yield from oxidation of β–hydroxybutyrate is: 26 ATP
49. Ketone bodies are utilised by: Extrahepatic tissue (Not by liver).
50. Causes for ketosis: Severe diabetes mellitus and starvation.
51. Ketogenesis is favoured by: High glucagon–insulin ratio.
52. Acetoacetate to β- hydroxy butyrate ratio depends on: NADH / NAD^+ ratio in mitochondria.

Metabolism of Unsaturated Fatty Acids and Eicosanoids

1. In human beings, enzymes can not introduce a double bond in a fatty acid beyond: Δ^9 Position.
2. The only polyunsaturated fatty acids which cannot be synthesised in the body are: Linoleic acid and linolenic acid.
3. Arachidonic acid can be formed from: Linoleic acid.
4. Monounsaturated fatty acids can be synthesised from saturated fatty acid by: Δ^9 desaturase enzyme system.
5. Energy yield in case of unsaturated fatty acids is: Less by 2 ATP molecules per double bond.
6. Energy yield from 1 molecule of palmitoelic acid (16 C monounsaturated) is: 127 ATP (129 – 2).
7. Prostanoids (Prostaglandins and thromboxanes) are formed by: Cyclooxygenase pathway.
8. The cyclooxygenase enzyme (prostaglandin synthase) is inhibited by: Nonsteroidal anti-inflammatory agents like aspirin, indomethacin and ibuprofen.
9. Rate limiting enzyme of prostaglandin synthesis is: phospholipase A_2 which hydrolyses phospholipids to liberate arachidonic acid.
10. Suicide enzyme is: Cyclooxygenase.
11. First prostaglandin to form is: PG – E_2.
12. Rate limiting enzyme of prostaglandin catabolic pathway is: 15–OH – PG – dehydrogenase.
13. Platelet aggregation is inhibited by: PGI_2
    Platelet aggregation is triggered by: TXA_2.
14. Prostaglandins are: Local hormones.
15. Leukotrienes and lipoxins are formed from: Lipoxygenase pathway.
16. Most potent chemotactic agent present in neutrophils is: LTB_4.
17. The slow reacting substance of anaphylaxis contains: LTC_4, LTD_4 and LTE_4.
18. Prolonged clotting time and low incidence of heart disease in eskimoes is due to: High intake of eicosapentanoic acid

Metabolism of Acylglycerols, Phospholipids and Sphingolipids

1. The major sites of triacylglycerol (TG) synthesis are: Liver and adipose tissue.
2. Triaclyglycerol is synthesized from: Free fatty acids and glycerol.
3. Glycerol part of fat is derived from: Metabolism of glucose.

4. Glycerol can not be directly used for esterification as adipose tissue lacks the enzyme: Glycerol kinase.
5. The products of lipolysis in adipose tissue are: Free fatty acids and glycerol.
6. Free fatty acids can be recycled for esterification by activation to acyl Co A by the enzyme: Acyl Co A synthase.
7. TG stores in the body are simultaneously undergoing: Lipolysis and reesterification.
8. TG in adipose tissue undergoes hydrolysis by: Hormone sensitive TG lipase.
9. TG from adipose tissue is mobilised under the effect of the hormones: glucagon and epinephrine.
10. Leptin is: A small peptides produced by adipocytes.
11. A defect in leptin or its receptor can lead to: Obesity.
12. Lipotropic factors are required for: Mobilization of fat from liver.
13. Deficiency of lipotropic factors lead to: Fatty liver.
14. Different lipotropic factors are: Choline, lecithin, methionine, betaine, inositol.
15. The metabolic precursor of phosphoglycerides is: Lysophosphatidate.
16. Glycerophospholipids with an ester linkage are synthesized from: Glycerol–3–PO_4.
17. The common precursor for synthesis of plasmalogens and platelet activating factor (phospholipids with ether linkages) is: Dihydroxy acetone phosphate.
18. Phospholipids are hydrolysed by enzymes: Phospholipases.
19. Most abundant phospholipids of cell membrane: Phosphatidylcholines.
20. Major phospholipids of cell membrane: Phosphoglyceride.
21. Basic structural unit of all sphingolipids is: Ceramide.
22. Sphingosine is formed from: Serine and palmitoyl CoA.
23. Sugars added to ceramide are first activated to: UDP linked sugar.
24. Diseases caused due to absence of enzymes degrading sphingolipids: Sphingolipidosis.

Metabolism of Lipoproteins

1. Lipoproteins serve as: Carrier of lipids in plasma.
2. Lipids need carrier for transport in plasma as: They are insoluble in water.
3. Lipoprotein complexes are made of:
   Hydrophobic lipids in core.
   Amphipathic lipids in outer layer
   Amphoproteins in outer most layer
4. TG formed in intestinal epithelial cells (exogenous TG) i.e. dietary TG is carried as: Chylomicrons.
5. Endogenous TG (TG formed in liver) is transported in plasma by: VLDL (very low density lipoprotein).

6. Fatty acids are made soluble by binding to: Albumin in plasma, Z- protein–in cells.
7. Main sites of metabolism of chylomicrons are: Adipose tissue and skeletal muscle.
8. Triacylglycerols of chylomicrons and VLDL are hydrolysed by: Lipoprotein lipase.
9. The enzyme lipoprotein lipase is located at: endothelial layer of capillaries of adipose tissue, muscles and heart.
10. Following injection of heparin, the lipoprotein lipase is released from the tissues and lipemia is thus cleared. This is called: Post heparin lipolytic activity.
11. Chylomicron formation fluctuates with: The load of TG absorbed.
12. The major apolipoprotein of chylomicrons is: Apo B_{48}.
13. The major apoporotein of LDL is: Apo B_{100}.
14. Degradation product of VLDL is: LDL through intermediate IDL.
15. Cholesterol is transported into the cell by: Endocytosis.
16. LDL receptors are located in specialized regions: Clathrin coated pits.
17. HDL is synthesized in: Liver.
18. Major apoprotein of HDL is: Apo–A.
19. The enzyme activity associated with HDL is: Lecithin cholesterol acyl transferase.
20. Longest single polypeptide chain is found in: Apo-B100 (4536 aminoacids).
21. Lipoprotein (*a*) is: Associated with myocardial infarction (Impairs fibrinolysis).
22. HDL–1 or HDL–C is: Hypercholesterolemic.
23. HDL–2 is involved in: Reverse cholesterol transport (inversely related to atherosclerosis).

Metabolism of cholesterol

1. Most common steroid in membrane is: Cholesterol
2. Storage form of cholesterol is: Cholesterol ester.
3. Source of cholesterol is by:
   (a) Dietary absorption
   (b) De novo synthesis.
4. Cholesterol is synthesized in: Endoplasmic reticulum and cytosol.
5. The amount of cholesterol synthesized per day is: 700 mg.
6. The carbon skeleton of cholesterol is derived from: Acetate moiety of acetyl CoA.
7. Rate limiting enzyme in cholesterol biosynthetic pathway is: HMG CoA reductase.
8. Immediate precursor sterol of cholesterol is: Lanosterol.
9. Hormonal effects on cholesterol biosynthesis: Insulin and thyroid hormones stimulate HMG CoA reductase activity while glucagon has opposite effect.
10. Site of absorption of cholesterol: First 100 cm of small intestine.
11. Drugs used to treat hypercholesterolemia are: Lovastatin and mevastatin.

12. The principal sterol excreted in faeces: Coprosterol.
13. Important compounds formed from cholesterol are:
    (a) Bile acids.
    (b) Steroid hormones
    (c) Vitamin D.
14. Primary bile acids are: Cholic acid and chenodeoxycholic acid.
15. Secondary bile acids are: Deoxycholic acid and lithocholic acid.
16. Rate limiting enzyme of bile acid synthesis is: 7α–hydroxylase.
17. Bile acid synthesis is affected by the deficiency of: Vitamin C.
18. Vitamin D is synthesised from: 7–dehydrocholesterol.

TABLE 1: Composition of Lipoprotein

	Chylo- microns	VLDL	IDL	LDL	HDL_2	HDL_3	FFA
Density (glml)	<0.95	0.95- 1.006	1.006- 1.019	1. 019- 1.063	1.063- 1.12	1.12- 1.21	1. 28- 1. 3
Diameter (nm)	75.- 1200	30- 80	15- 35	18- 25	10- 12	7,5- - 10	
Origin	Intestine	Liver VLDLs	VL v+DLs	VLDLs IDLs/Liver	Intestine and Liver	Liver &	Adipose tissue
Electrophoretic mobility	Origin	Per-β	Per–β	β or β	α		Albumin
Composition (%)							
Triacylglycerol	86	52	28	10	10	5	0
Cholesteryl ester	3	14	30	38	21	14	0
Free cholesterol	1	7	8	8	7	3	0
Phospholipid	8	18	23	22	29	19	0
Protein	2	8	11	21	33	57	99
FFA	0	0	0	0	0	0	1
Apoproteins	A, B-48, C-II, E	B-100 C-II, E	B-100 E	B-100	AI-C,	E	Albumin
Transport function	TAG	TAG		Choles- terol	Cholesterol		FFA
Transport from	Gut	Liver	LDL precursor	Liver	Reverse cholesterol		Adipose tissue
To	Muscle & adipose tissue	muscle		Periphe- ral	Transport system tissue		Muscle & Liver

TABLE 2: Apoproteins of human Plasma Lipoproteins

Apoprotein	Mol. wt	Lipoprotein	Functions
Apo A–I	28,000	Chylomicrons, HDL–2	Reversecholesterol transport, Activator of lecithin:cholesterolacyl transferase (LCAT) ligand for HDL receptor
Apo A–II	17,000	Chylomicrons, HDL–3	Inhibitor of apo A-I and LCAT, stimulates lupatic lipase
Apo B–100	5,12,000	VLDL ,IDL ,LDL	Ligand for LDL receptor
Apo B–48	2,64,000	Chylomicrons	48% size of B-100 hence the name chylomicron secretion from intestine
Apo C – I	7000	Chylomicrons VLDL, HDL	Activation of LCAT
Apo C – II	9000	Chylomicrons VLDL, HDL	Activates extrahepatic lipoprotein lipase
Apo C – III	9000	Chylomicrons VLDL, HDL	Inhibits lipoprotein lipase, antiatherogenic
Apo D	19,300	HDL–3	Lipid transfer protein
Apo E	38,00	Chylomicrons VLDL,IDL HDL	Arginine rich ligand for chylomicron remnant receptor in liver and LDL receptor.

TABLE 3: Classification of Hyperlipoproteinemia

Type fraction elevated	Lipoprotein	Cholesterol Level	TG Level	Metabolic defect
Type I Rare autosomal recessive	(a) Chylomicrons (b) VLDL ↑ in Case of ↑ carbohydarate intake	N	↑↑	(i) Lipoprotein lipase deficiency autosomal case of ↑ (ii) A variant can be produced by apoC – II deficiency
Type II A common autosomal dominant	LDL	↑↑	N	(i) LDL receptor deficiency common (ii) Defective binding of B-100 Autosomal to the receptor (iii) Receptor-LDL complex not-dominant internalised properly
Type II B	LDL and VLDL	↑↑	↑	Excess of apo B
Type III Autosomal Dominant tranferase	Broad-β (IDL), VLDL and Chylomicrons	↑	↑	(i) Abnormal apo-E concentration(↑) (ii) ↑ synthesis of apo-B
Type IV Autosomal Dominant	VLDL	N ↑	↑	↑ Endogenous synthesis of TG ↓Catabolism of both
Type V Autosomal Dominant	Chylomicron and VLDL	N	↑	Secondary to other causes obesity, excess alcohol intake, renal failure, Pancreatitis

TABLE 4: Hypolipoproteinemia				
Disease	**Lipoproteins**	**Cholesterol**	**TG**	**Clinical findings**
(1) Familial hypobeta lippoproteinemia	LDL ↓ B – 100 ↓	↓	N	↓ risk of CAD
(2) Abetali-poproteinemia	VLDL ↓ LDL ↓↓ B-48 ↓ B-100 ↓↓	Markedly Decreased	↓	Malabsorption Physical & mental retardation, fatty infiltration acanthocytosis
(3) Hypoalpha Lipoproteinemia	HDL ↓ A–I ↓	N	N	↑ risk of CAD
(4) Familial α lipoprotein deficiency	HDL ↓↓ Apo–A I ↓↓	N	N	↑ risk of CAD

TABLE: 5 Sphingolipidoses (Lipid Storage Diseases)			
No.	**Disease**	**Enzyme defect**	**Lipid accumulation**
1	Gaucher's disease	β- Glucosidase	Glucocerebroside
2	Niemann–Pick disease	Sphingomyelinase	Sphingomyelin
3	Krabbe's Leukodystrophy	β-Galactosidase	Galactocerebroside
4	Metachromatic Leukodystrophy	Sulfatide sulfatase	Sulfogalactocerebroside
5	Fabr'y disease	α-Galactosidase	Ceramide trinexoside
6	Tay–sachs disease	Hexaminidase A	Ganglioside (GM2)
7	Generalized gangliosidoses	β-Gaiactosidase	Ganglioside (GM1)
8	Lactosyl ceramidoses	β-Galactosidase	Lactosyl ceramide
9	Sand Hoff's disease	Hexosaminidase A and B	Globoside

SOLVED QUESTIONS

Q.1. The most essential fatty acid is: (AIPGME 1995)

1. **Linoleic acid**
2. **Linolenic acid**
3. **Arachidonic acid**
4. **Palmitic acid.**

Ans. 1

Linoleic acid, linolenic acid and arachidonic acid are the three essential fatty acid. Among these the most essential fatty acid is linoleic acid because arachidonic acid is synthesised from linoleic acid by a three stage reaction. Biologically arachidonic acid is important as it is a precursor of prostaglandins and leukotrienes.

Q.2. The most imprtant carrier of cholesterol in plasma is: (AIPGME 1997)

1. **Chylomicrons**
2. **HDL**
3. **VLDL**
4. **LDL.**

Ans. 4

The LDL molecules are cholesterol rich (46% in composition) lipoproteins molecules. About 75% of the plasma cholesterol is incorporated into the LDL particles. Chylomicrons are rich in triglycerides (83% composition). They transport exogenous triglcyerides from gut to muscle and adipose tissue.

VLDL are the major carriers of endogenous triglycerides.

HDL transport cholesterol from peripheral tissues to liver.

Q.3. Endogenous triglycerides in plasma are maximally carried in: (AIPGME 1998)

1. **VLDL**
2. **Chylomicrons**
3. **LDL**
4. **HDL**

Ans. 1

VLDL molecules are the major carriers of endogenous triglycerides. They are synthesised in the liver from glycerol and fatty acids and incorporated into VLDL. Exogenous triglyceride (dietary TG) is transported by chylomicrons. Chylomicrons are formed in the intestinal mucosal cells

LDL molecules transport cholesterol from liver to the peripheral tissues.

HDL transport cholesterol from peripheral tissues to liver.

Q.4. Dietary cholesterol is delivered transported to extra hepatic tissue by: (AIPGME 1999)

1. **VLDL**
2. **LDL**
3. **Chylomicrons**
4. **IDL**

Ans. 2

[Explanation same as Q.2]

IDL is VLDL remnant and it is further converted to LDL.

Q.5. All of the following statements are true regarding lipoproteins except: (AIPGME 2001)

1. **VLDL transports endogenous lipids**
2. **LDL transports lipids to the tissues.**
3. **Increased blood cholesterol is associated with increased LDL receptors**
4. **Increased HDL is associated with decreased risk of coronary disease**

Ans. 3

The primary function of LDL particles is to provide cholesterol to the peripheral tissues. Specific receptors for LDL are present on the cell surface membranes. These receptors recognize Apo B-100 of LDL. After binding , the LDL is internalized by endocytosis. Deficiency of functional LDL receptors causes a significant rise in plasma LDL i.e. in plasma cholesterol.

Q.6. Which of these fatty acids is found exclusively in breast milk? (AIPGME 2001)

1. **Linoleate**
2. **Linolenic**
3. **Palmitic**
4. **Docosahexaenoic acid.**

Ans. 4

Docosahexaenoic acid (DHA) which is a very long chain fatty acid is synthesized from ∝-linolenic acid or directly obtained from fish oils. It is present in high concentrations in retina cerebral cortex, testis and sperm. DHA is required for brain and retina development and is supplied via the placenta and milk . Milk is the constant and continuous source of DHA as placenta is not present at all time

Q.7. Dietary triglycerides are transported by: (AIIMS May 2001)

1. **Chylomicrons**
2. **VLDL**
3. **LDL**
4. **HDL.**

Ans. 1

Explanation same as Q.3.

Q.8. Bile acids are derived from: (AIPGME 1994)

1. **Fatty acids**
2. **Cholesterol**
3. **Bilirubin**
4. **Proteins.**

Ans. 2

More than 50% cholesterol is converted to bile acids and excreted in faeces. Primary bile acids are synthesised from cholesterol in the liver by using molecular O_2, NADPH, and cytochrome P-450.

Q.9. NADPH is used in: (AIPGME 1995)

1. **Fatty acid synthesis**

2. **Ketone synthesis**
3. **Gluconeogenesis**
4. **Glycolysis**

Ans. 1

Q.10. NADPH is required for **(AIPGME 1998)**

1. **Gluconeogenesis**
2. **Glycolysis**
3. **Fatty acid synthesis**
4. **Glycogenolysis**

Ans. 3

NADPH is required for reductive biosynthetic reactions eg. de novo synthesis of fatty acid, synthesis of cholesterol, synthesis of bile acids. NADPH is generated mainly by the HMP shunt pathway. For reducing reactions in catabolic pathways NADH is used .

Q.11. Rate limiting enzyme in the synthesis of cholesterol is: **(AJPG 1995)**

1. **HMG CoA reductase**
2. **HMG CoA synthetase**
3. **Acetyl CoA synthetase**
4. **Acetyl CoA carboxylase**

Ans. 1

Rate limiting enzyme in the cholesterol synthesis is HMG CoA reductase. (3-Hydroxy-3- methylglutaryl Co A reductase). Reductase activity is reduced by fasting and by cholesterol feeding and thus provides effective feed back control of cholesterol metabolism. It catalyses the conversion of HMG CoA to mevalonate.

Q.12. Apoprotein A is found in: **(AIPGME 1996)**

1. **Chylomicrons**
2. **VLDL**
3. **HDL**
4. **LDL.**

Ans. 3

Apoprotein A is major apoprotein of HDL. The apo A-I of HDL activates LCAT (Lecithin Cholesterol Acyl Transferase) present in the plasma. The LCAT then binds to the HDL disc. Mature HDL spheres are taken up by liver cells by apo-A- I mediated receptor mechanism. Chylomicrons – contain only apo B-48 and apo A but apo-C and apo-E are added from serum

VLDL has–Apo B-100, C-II and E

LDL has only apo B-100

Q.13. The first step in fatty acid synthesis involves: (AIPGME 1996)

1. **Acetyl CoA carboxylase**
2. **β-hydroxyl CoA dehydrogenase**
3. **Acetyl dehydrogenase**
4. **Pyruvate kinase.**

Ans. 1

The first step in fatty acid synthesis is the carboxylation of acetyl CoA to form malonyl CoA with the help of enzyme acetyl CoA carboxylase. It is the rate limiting enzyme. Pyruvate kinase is an enzyme of glycolysis.

Q.14. Gauchers disease is due to deficiency of enzyme: (AIPGME 1999)

1. **Sphingomyelinase**
2. **β-Glucosidase**
3. **Hexosaminidase - A**
4. **β-galactosidase.**

Ans. 2

The defective enzyme in Gaucher's disease is β-glucosidase, leading to abormality in the catabolism of glucocerebrosides (Glycosphingolipid)

Glucocerebroside β-glucosidase → Ceramide + glucose

Absence of this enzyme results in the accumulation of glucocerebroside. Hexosaminidase-A catalyses GM_2 catabolism. Sphingomyelinase catalyses sphingomyelin catabolism. β-galactosidase is associated with galactocerebroside catabolism.

Q.15. Which helps in the transport of chylomicrons from intestine to liver: (AIPGME 2000)

1. **Apoprotein B**
2. **Apoprotein A**
3. **Apoprotein C**
4. **Apoprotein E.**

Ans. 1

Chylomicrons have 3 apoproteins – Apo B-48, Apo C, and ApoE. Chylomicrons are assembled in intestinal mucosal cells. When they are released from intestine, they have only one apoprotein Apo B-48 and are called nascent chylomicrons. In the circulation chylomicrons receive Apo C and Apo E from circulating HDL. Apo C-II of chylomicron particles activate lipoprotein lipase in peripheral tissues and adipose tissue. After this Apo C-II return to HDL. The chylomicron remnants are then taken up by hepatocytes . The receptor binds with Apo-E and then chylomicrons are taken up. Thus the only apoprotien associated with chylomicrons during its transport from intestine to liver is Apo B-48.

Q.16. In a well fed state, acetyl CoA obtained from diet is least used in the synthesis of: (AIPGME 2002)

1. **Palmityl CoA**
2. **Citrate**
3. **Acetoacetate**
4. **Oxalosuccinate.**

Ans. **3**

Acetoacetate is a ketone body. Ketone body metabolism is increased during starvation or diabetic ketoacidosis. In starvation, the dietary supply of glucose is decreased . The increased rate of lipolysis is to provide alternate source of fuel. The excess acetyl CoA is converted to ketone bodies. But in a well fed state, as glucose is available, acetyl CoA is chanelled through TCA cycle and used for energy production.Citrate and oxalosuccinate are intermediates of TCA cycle. Some acetyl CoA is used for synthesis of fatty acid (palmityl CoA). While acetyl CoA is least used for ketone body production.

Q.17. β-oxidation of odd chain fatty acids produces: (AIPGME 2003)

1. **Succinyl CoA**
2. **Propionyl CoA**
3. **Acetyl CoA**
4. **Malonyl CoA.**

Ans. **2**

β-oxidation of odd chain fatty acids after successive removal of 2- carbon units, at the end produces one 3 carbon unit, propionyl CoA.

Q.18. A person on a fat free carbohydrate rich diet continues to grow obese, which of the following lipoproteins is likely to be elevated in his blood ?(AIPGME 2004)

1. **Chylomicrons**
2. **VLDL**
3. **LDL**
4. **HDL.**

Ans. **2**

The person is on a fat free diet so chylomicron synthesis (exogenous TG transporter) is not seen. But as the diet is rich in carbohydrate there is increased synthesis of glycerol and fatty acids. They are incorporated into VLDL along with hepatic, cholesterol, apo- B-100. C-II and E. This leads to elevated VLDL levels in the blood .

Q.19. Acetyl-CoA acts as a substrate for all the enzyme except: (AIIMS May 2003)

1. **HMG CoA synthetase**
2. **Malic enzyme**
3. **Malonyl CoA synthetase**
4. **Fatty acid synthetase.**

Ans. **2**

Except malic enzyme, rest all the three enzyme uses acetyl CoA as a substrate. Malic enzyme catalyses the oxidative decarboxylation of cytoplasmic malate

Malate + $NADP^+$ + Malic enzyme → Pyruvate +Co_2+ NADPH + H^+.

Q.20. Which of the following is increased in lipoprotein lipase deficiency: (AIIMS May 2001)

1. **VLDL**
2. **LDL**
3. **HDL**
4. **Chylomicrons.**

Ans. **4**

Type	Primary disease	Basic defect	Elevated lipoprotein
I	Familial lipoprotein lipase deficiency	Lipoprotein lipase deficiency	Chylomicrons
II a	Familial Hypercholesterolemia	LDL receptor defect	LDL
II b	Familial mixed lipoproteinemia	Excess of apo B	LDL and VLDL
III	Familial type III Hyperlipoproteinemia	Abnormal apo E	Chylomicron remnants and IDL
IV	Familial triglyceridemia	Overproduction of VLDL	VLDL
V	Familial combined hyperlipidemia	Deficiency of apo-C	VLDL, chylomicrons

Q.21. Accumulation of sphingomyelin in phagocytic cells is feature of: (AIIMS Nov 2002)

1. **Gaucher's disease**
2. **Niemann pick disease**
3. **Tay sach's disease**
4. **Down's syndrome**

Ans. **2**

Disease	Enzyme defect	Lipid Accumulating
(1) Gaucher's disease	b-glucosidase	Glucocerebroside
(2) Niemann-pick disease	Sphingomyelinase	Sphingomyelin
(3) Krabbe's leukodystrophy	b-galactosidase	Galactocerebroside
(4) Metachromatic leukodystrophy	Sulfatide sulfatase	Sulfogalactocerebroside
(5) Fabry's disease	a-galactosidase	Ceramide trihexoside
(6) Tay-sach's disease	Hexosaminidase A	Ganglioside (Gm_2)
(7) Generalised gangliosidoses	Beta-galactosidase	Ganglioside (GM_1)
(8) Lactosyl ceramidoses	Beta-galactosidase	Lactosyl ceramide

Q.22. In synthesis of fatty acids energy is supplied by: (AIIMS May 2002)

1. **NAD**
2. **FAD**
3. **GTP**
4. **NADPH**

Ans. 4

Fatty acid synthesis is a reductive biosynthetic reaction so the reducing equivalents are provided by NADPH

Q.23. Choesterol present in LDL: (AIIMS May 2003)

1. **Represents primarily cholesterol that is being removed from peripheral cell**
2. **Binds to a receptor and diffuses across the cell membrane**
3. **On accumlation in the cell inhibits replenishment of LDL receptors**
4. **When enters a cell, suppresses activity of acyl CoA: cholesterol acyltransferase (ACAT)**

Ans. 3

LDL delivers cholesterol to extrahepatic tissue so does not represent cholesterol removed from peripheral cells Apo B-100 of LDL binds to specific receptor on cell membrane.

When delivered in the cells, cholesterol is stored as cholesterol esters after esterification catalysed by ACAT. When intracellular cholesterol level increases, its accumulation wihtin the cell inhibits the synthesis of new LDL receptors.

Q.24. All of the following statements about LDL are true except: (AIIMS may 2004)

1. **It delivers cholesterol to cells**
2. **It contains only one Apoprotein**
3. **It is a marker for cardiovascular disease**
4. **It contains Apo-B4**

Ans. 4

LDL molecules are cholesterol rich lipoproteins. They transport the cholesterol from liver to peripheral tissues. The only apoprotein present on LDL is Apo B-100. LDL concentration in blood has positive correlation with incidence of cardiovascular disease so it is a marker for cardiovascular disease.

Q.25. The most imprtant source of reducing equivalents for fatty acid synthesis in the liver is: (AIIMS May 2004)

1. **Glycolysis**
2. **TCA cycle**
3. **Uronic acid pathway**
4. **HMP pathway**

Ans. 4

Fatty acid synthesis involves reductive biosynthetic reactions for which reducing equivalents are provided by NADPH. HMP pathway provides NADPH.

During reducing reactions in catabolic pathways like glycolysis, TCA cycle and uronic acid pathway NADH is produced

Q.26. Apo B_{48} and Apo B_{100} are expressed as two different apoproteins because of difference in: (AIPGME 2002)

1. **RNA editing**
2. **RNA splicing**
3. **Chromosomal loci**
4. **Apo-B gene.**

Ans. 1

Apo B_{48} and apo B_{100} are the products of the same gene, but in intestine, the mRNA undergoes editing so as to produce B-48 protein. The codon at 2153 (CAA) is changed to a stop codon by an 'RNA editing' mechanism (deamination of cytosine to uracil). Apo B_{48} is 48 % size of B_{100}; hence the name. Therefore, Apo B_{48} and apo B_{100} differ due to the RNA editing occurring in the intestinal cells.

Q.27. To which of the following family of chemical mediators of inflammation the lipoxins belong:

1. **Kinin system**
2. **Cytokines**
3. **Chemokines**
4. **Arachidonic acid metabolites**

Ans. 4

Lipoxins are a group of compounds produced by leukocytes . They are conjugated tetraenes. They are formed by sequential action of 5 and 15 lipo oxygenases. L_XA_4 is the most common variety. It is chemotactic.

Q.28. Unsaturated fatty acids are converted to:

1. **Prostaglandins**
2. **Cholesterol**
3. **Cell membrane lipid**
4. **Saturated fatty acid**

Ans. 1

Animal tissues have limited capacity for desaturating fatty acids and that process requires certain dietary polyunsaturated fatty acids derived from plants. These essential fatty acids are used to form eicosanoic fatty acids which in turn give rise to the prostaglandins and thromboxanes and to leukotrienes and lipoxins - known collectively as eicosanoids.

Q.29. Oxidation of fatty acid occur in:

1. **Cytoplasm**
2. **Ribosomes**
3. **Centrioles**
4. **Mitochondria**

Ans. 4

Acyl COA synthetase required for the β -oxidation of fatty acids are found in the endoplasmic reticulum, peroxisomes, and inside and on the outer membrane of mitochondria.

Q.30. Rate limiting step in cholesterol synthesis is:

1. **HMG CoA synthetase**
2. **HMG CoA lyase**
3. **HMG CoA reductase**
4. **Mevalonate synthetase**

Ans. 3

Acetoacetyl COA condenses with acetyl COA in presence of HMG-COA synthase to form HMG-COA, which is reduced to mevalonate by NADPH catalyzed by HMG-COA reductase. This is the principal regulatory step in the pathway of cholesterol synthesis and is the site of action of the most effective class of cholesterol-lowering drugs, the HMG COA reductase inhibitors (Statins1).

Q.31. Ketone body which is maximum in diabetic ketoacidosis:

1. **Acetone**
2. **Pyruvate**
3. **Acetocetic acid**
4. **β-oxaloacetate**

Ans. 3

Acetoacetic acid and 3-Hydroxybutyric acids are both moderately strong acids and are buffered when present in blood or other tissues. However, their continual excretion in quantity progressively depletes the alkali reserve, causing keto acidosis. This may be fatal in uncontrolled diabetes mellitus.

Q.32. Limiting factor for Fatty acid synthesis:

1. **Acetoacetate synthetase**
2. **Acyl transferase**
3. **Acetyl COA carboxylase**
4. **Biotin**

Ans. 3

Acetyl COA carboxylase is an allosteric enzyme and is activated by citrate, citrate converts the enzyme from an inactive dimer to an active polymeric form, having a molecular mass of sevaral million. Inactivation is promoted by phosphorylation of the enzyme and by long chain acyl COA molecules, an example of negative feedback inhibition by a product of a reaction. Thus if acyl COA accumulates because it is not esterified quickly enough or because of increased lipolysis or an influx of free fatty acids into the tissues, it will automatically reduce the synthesis of new fatty acids.

Q.33. The sugar component of cerebrosides is:

1. **Fructose**
2. **Sucrose**
3. **Galactose**
4. **Glucose**

Ans. 3, 4

The cerebrosides are galactosylceramide (Gal.cer) and glucosylceramide (Glc.cer.) Gal-cer is a major lipid of myelin, whereas Glc.cer is a major glycosphingolipid of extraneural tissues and a precursor of most of the more complex glycosphingolipids.

Q.34. Endogenous triglycerides in plasma is maximally bound to:

1. **Chylomicrons**
2. **LDL**
3. **VLDL**
4. **HDL**

Ans. 3

VLDL's are the vehicles of transport of triacylglycerol from the liver to the extrahepatic tissues.

Q.35. The substance essential for transfer of fatty acids across mitochondrial membrane:

1. **Creatine**
2. **Creatinine**
3. **Carnitine**
4. **Coenzyme A**

Ans. 3

Long chain acyl COA or (FFA) will not penetrate the inner membrane of mitochondria. However, carnitine palmitocyltransferase- I, present in the outer mitochondrial membrane, converts, long chain acyl COA to acylcarnitine, which is able to penetrate the inner membrane and gain access to the β-oxidation system of enzyme.

Q.36. One of the following is a scavenger of cholesterol from tissue and prevents atherosclerosis:

1. **VLDL**
2. **LDL**
3. **Chylomicrons**
4. **HDL**

Ans. 4

HDL concentration are inversely related to the incidence of coronary atherosclerosis, possibly because they reflect the efficiency of reverse cholesterol transport.

Q.37. Ganglioside is composed of all except:

1. **Galactose**
2. **Phosphate**
3. **Ceramide**
4. **Sialic acid.**

Ans. 2

Gangliosides are complex glycosphingolipids derived from glucosylceramide that contains in addition one or more molecules of sialic acid.

Q.38. Gaucher's disease is due to the accumulation of:

1. **Glucose**
2. **Galactose**
3. **Glucocerebroside**
4. **Sphingomyelin.**

Ans. 3

Gaucher's disease is caused due to the deficiency of enzyme β-glucosidase to which there is a accumulation of glucosylceramide and shows enlargement of liver and spleen, erosion of long bones, and mental retardation in infants.

Q.39. "Squalene" is the intermediate product during synthesis of:

1. **VLDL**
2. **Cholesterol**
3. **Tachysterol**
4. **Ionosterol**

Ans. 2

Squalene is formed from six isoprenoid units. It cyclizes to give rise to parent steroid ionosterol from which cholesterol is formed.

Q.40. The lipid which accumulates in fatty liver is:

1. **Triglycerides**
2. **FFA**
3. **Lipoprotein**
4. **Cholesterol**

Ans. 1

Lipids mainly as triacyl glycerol can accumulate in the liver and causes fatty liver.

Q.41. Apolipoprotein activating L-CAT:

1. **B-48**

2. A-I
3. A-II
4. B-100

Ans. 2

LCAT- Lecithin cholesterol acyl transferase is a plasma enzyme. This is similar to the lipoproteins and can be activated by Apo A-I

Q.42. Prostaglandin synthesis is partially switched off by:

1. Lipoxygenase inhibition
2. Cyclo-oxygenase inhibition
3. Reductase
4. Peroxidase

Ans. 2

Arachidonate, is the substrate for the synthesis of the PG2, TX2 series (prostanoids) by the cyclooxygenases and when aspirin, a nonsteroidal anti-inflammatory drug (NSAID) inhibits cyclooxygenases competing with arachidonate. prostaglandin synthesis is automatically switched off.

Q.43. Ketone bodies are by products of metabolism of:

1. Carbohydrate
2. Protein
3. Fat
4. All of the above

Ans. 3

Free fatty acids are the precursors of ketone bodies in the liver.

Q.44. Maple syrup urine disease is due to deficiency of:

1. Decarboxylation of keto acids
2. Hydroxylation
3. Methylation
4. None of the above

Ans. 1

The odor of urine in maple syrup urine disease suggests maple syrup or burnt sugar. This biochemical defect involves the ∝- keto acid decarboxylase complex.

Q.45. Fredrickson's type II hyperlipoproteinemia is due to excess amounts of:

1. VLDL remnants
2. VLDL
3. Floating LDL
4. HDL

Ans. **3**

Type II hyperlipoproteinemia is caused due to the defective LDL receptors or mutation in ligand region of apo B-100. The disease shows the elevated levels of LDL and hypercholesterolemia resulting in atherosclerosis and coronary disease.

Q.46. Triglyceride synthesis is increased by:

1. **Growth hormone**
2. **Insulin**
3. **Cortisol**
4. **Glucagon**

Ans. **2**

Insulin inhibits the release of free fatty acids from adipose tissue, which is followed by a fall in circulating plasma free fatty acids. It enhances lipogenesis and the synthesis of acylglycerol and increase the oxidation of glucose to CO_2 via pentose phosphate pathway.

Q.47. The substance which accumulates in Tay Sach's disease is:

1. **Cerebroside**
2. **Ganglioside**
3. **Sphingosine**
4. **Sphingomyelin**

Ans. **2**

Tay sach's disease is caused dut ot the deficiency of the enzyme hexosaminidase A. During this disease there is an accumulation of gangliosides and the symptoms include mental retardation, blindness and muscular weakness.

Q.48. Which has the highest cholesterol content?

1. **HDL**
2. **LDL**
3. **VLDL**
4. **Chylomicron**

Ans. **2**

LDL contains the cholesterol as the main lipid component.

Q.49. Chymotrypsinogen is a: **(AIIMS Nov 2006)**

1. **Zymogen.**
2. **Carboxypeptidase.**
3. **Transaminase.**
4. **Elastase.**

Ans. **1**

Chymotrypsinogen is a zymogen. Zymogens are inactive precursors of secreted enzymes (including the proteases required for digestion). They become activated through cleavage when they reach their proper sites of action. For example the pancreatic zymogen, trypsinogen, becomes activated to trypsin in the small intestine. This activated trypsin can than activate chymotrypsinogen to chymotrypsin, proelastase to elastase, procarboxypeptidase to carboxypeptidase, and proaminopeptidase to aminopeptidase.

Q.50. High levels of lipoprotein (a) is most likely to be associated with: (AIIMS Nov 2006)

1. **Atherosclerosis.**
2. **Cirrhosis.**
3. **Renal failure.**
4. **Pancreatitis.**

Ans. 1

Lipoprotein (a) consists of 1 mole of LDL attached to 1 mole of apoA, which shows structural homology to plasminogen hence it inhibits fibrinolysis and favours atherosclerosis. High levels of lipoprotein (a) may leads to premature coronary heart disease due to atherosclerosis and thrombosis due to inhibition of fibrinolysis.

Q.51. Eicosapentaenoic acid is present in: (AIIMS Nov 2006)

5. **Fish oil.**
6. **Soya bean oil.**
7. **Corn oil.**
8. **Cod liver oil.**

Ans. 1

Eicosapentaenoic acid is a fatty acid with 20-carbon atom and 5 double bonds and it is a ω_3 fatty acid also called as timnodonic acid.

When it is present with 20 carbon atoms and 4 double bonds then it is ω_6 fatty acid. Now this is called as arachidonic acid and is found in animal fats.

Q.52. The human plasma lipoprotein containing the highest percentage of triacylglycerols by weight is: (AIPGEE 2006)

1. **VLDL.**
2. **Chylomicrons.**
3. **HDL.**
4. **LDL.**

Ans. 2

Chylomicrons are the lipoprotein particles lowest in density and largest in size, and contain the highest percentage of lipid and the smallest percentage of protein. VLDL's and LDL's are successively denser, having higher ratios of protein to lipid. HDL particle are the densest.

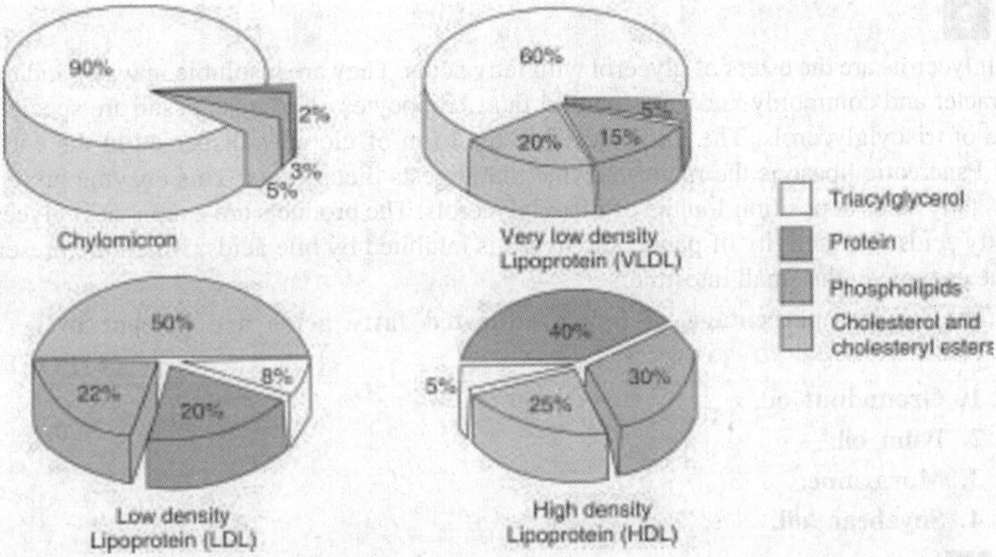

Fig.3.1. Composition of the plasma lipoproteins. Note high concentration of cholesterol and cholesteryl estersin LDL.

Q.53. The ligand receptor complex dissociates in the endosome because: (AIPGEE 2006)

1. **Of its large size.**
2. **The vesicle looses its clathrin coat.**
3. **Of the acidic pH of the vesicle.**
4. **Of the basic pH of the vesicle.**

Ans. 3

The ligand receptor complex dissociates into the endosome due to the acidic pH of the vesicle. The best example of ligand receptor complex is LDL receptor-Apo B_{100}.

LDL receptors are negatively charged glycoproteins that are clustered in pits on cell membranes. The intracellular side of the pit is coated with the protein clathrin, which stabilizes the shape of the pit. After binding, the LDL receptor complex is internalized by endocytosis. The vesicle containing the LDL rapidly loses its clathrin coat and fuses with other smaller vesicles, forming larger vesicles called endosomes. The pH of the endosomes falls due to the proton pumping activity of endosomal ATPase, this allows the separation of the LDL from its receptor. The receptor then migrates to one side of the endosome, whereas the LDL's stay free within the lumen of the vesicle.

Q.54. Regarding triacylglycerol metabolism in adipocytes all are true except: (AIPGEE 2007)

1. **Storage forms of lipid in body.**
2. **Glycerol kinase.**
3. **Metabolized by lipoprotein lipase.**
4. **Metabolism of triacylglycerol is inhibited by bile acids.**

Ans. **2**

Triacylglycerols are the esters of glycerol with fatty acids. They are insoluble in water and non polar in character and commonly known as neutral fats. Adipocytes of adipose tissue are specialized for storage of triacylglycerols. The fat is stored in the form of globules dispersed in the entire cytoplasm. Pancreatic lipase is the major enzyme that digests dietary fats. This enzyme preferentially cleaves fatty acids at position 1 and 3 of triacylglycerols. The products are 2 monoacyl glycerols and free fatty acids. The activity of pancreatic lipase is inhibited by bile acids, which are present along with the enzyme in the small intestine.

Q.55. The highest percentage of polyunsaturated fatty acids are present in?

(AIPGEE 2007)

1. **Groundnut oil.**
2. **Palm oil.**
3. **Margraine.**
4. **Soyabean oil.**

Ans. **4**

Some polyunsaturated fatty acids eg. linoleic acid, a-linoleic acid is found in high concentrations in vegetable oils and in small amounts in animal carcasses.

4

Proteins

1. The chemical nature and structure of different amino acids are defined by: Side chain (R).
2. The only optically inactive amino acid is: Glycine.
3. An α–amino acid is the one in which: Both the amino and carbonyl group are attached to the same 'C'atom i.e. α – carbon.
4. Classification of amino acids:
   (a) Based on nature of side chain:
      (i) Aliphatic amino acids (aliphatic nonpolar side chains)–Glycine, alanine, valine, leucine, isoleucine.
      (ii) Aromatic amino acids – Phenylalanine, tyrosine, tryptophan, histidine.
      (iii) Hydroxyl containing amino acids – Serine, threonine, tyrosine.
      (iv) Acidic amino acids and amides - Aspartate, asparagine, glutamate, glutamine.
      (v) Basic amino acids–Lysine, histidine, arginine.
      (vi) Sulfur containing amino acids–Cysteine, methionine.
      (vii) Imino acid – Proline.
   (b) According to solubitity of side chain:
      (i) Hydrophilic – Glycine, glutamine, glutamic acid, aspartic acid, asparagine, histidine, arginine, cysteine, serine, threonine, lysine.
      (ii) Hydrophobic – Alanine, valine, leucine, isoleucine, phenylalanine, tyrosine, tryptophan, methionine, proline.
   (c) According to dietary requirement:
      (i) Essential amino acids (Indispensable amino acids) – Phenylalanine, tryptophan, threonine, lysine, leucine, isoleucine, methionine and valine.
      (ii) Partially essential (Semi- indispensable) amino acids – Histidine, arginine.
      (iii) Nonessential (Dispensable amino acid)– All others.

(d) Based on metabolic fate:
Ketogenic amino acid – Leucine. Partially ketogenic and partially glucogenic-Lysine, isoleucine, phenylalanine tyrosine and tryptophan. Glucogenic amino acids – All others.

5. Naturally occuring amino acids are: L – α – amino acid.
6. An L – α – amino acids has spatial configuration similar to: L – Glyceraldehydes.
7. Amino acids in neutral solution are dipolar in charge (no net charge) and are called: Zwitterion.
8. Amino acid with pk value within physiological range of pH: Histidine (pk=6.0).
9. Most basic amino acid: Arginine.
10. Amino acid containing indole ring: Tryptophan.
11. Amino acid deficient in maize are: Tryptophan and lysine.
12. Amino acid absent in wheat: Lysine.
13. Amino acid not found in bean: Methionine.
14. Most of U.V. light absorption of proteins above 240 nm is due to: Aromatic amino acid (Tryptophan).
15. Phosphorylation of enzymes during their regulation by cAMP is initiated at: Serine, threonine or tyrosine (–OH containing amino acids).
16. Majority of total body amino acids are generated by: Muscles.
17. All amino acids undergo transamination except: Lysine, threonine, proline, hydroxyproline.
18. The only amino acid in humans that can undergo oxidative deamination considerably: L – glutamate.
19. The amino acids in peptides and proteins are linked by: Peptide bond.
20. The nature of peptide bond is: Partial double bond.

Colour Reactions of Proteins

	Test	Group responsible	Compounds giving positive test	Remarks
1.	Biuret	More than one peptide bond	Tri–oligo; polypeptides proteins	Amino acids and dipeptides do not give this test
2.	Ninhydrin	α-amino group	α-amino acids	Proline and OH-proline do not give this test
3.	Xantho proteic	Benzene ring	Aromatic amino acids	--
4.	Millon's	Phenolic group	Tyrosine	--
5.	Cole's aldehyde	Indole	Tryptophan	Gelatin and collagen do not give this test
6.	Lead acetate	Sulphur containing amino acid	Cysteine and Cystine	Methionine does not give this test
7.	Sakaguchi	Guanidino	Arginine	--

21. Classification of proteins:
    A. According to shape–
        (i) Fibrous – Axial ratio > 10
        (ii) Globular – Axial ratio < 10
    B. Based on functions–
        (i) Catalytic proteins (Enzymes) – Trypsin, pepsin etc.
        (ii) Contractile proteins – Actin, myosin.
        (iii) Gene regulatory proteins – Histones, repressor proteins.
        (iv) Hormonal role - Insulin.
        (v) Protective role - Immunoglobulins, interferon,
        (vi) Regulatory proteins – Calmodulin.
        (vii) Structural proteins – Collagen, elastin, keratins.
        (viii) Transport Proteins-Albumin (for bilirubin, fatty acids, some hormones etc), hemoglobin (O_2, CO_2), lipoproteins (insoluble lipids, fat soluble vitamins), transferrin (iron).
22. Primary structure of protein is: Total number and amino acid sequence that specifies 3 dimensional structure.
23. Secondary structure denotes: The configurational relationship between 'residues which are about 3-4 amino acids apart in linear sequence.
24. Tertiary structure of protein refers to: Steric relationship of amino acids close to one another in amino acid sequence.
25. Quaternary structure of protein is: Manner in which subunits are packed together.
26. Pitch of alpha helix of proteins is about: 0.54 nm.
27. The $\propto$-helix is generally right handed because amino acids found in protein are of: L-variety.
28. The amino acids residues destabilizing the $\propto$–helix formation: Arginine, aspartic acid, glutamic acid, lysine.
29. The amino acids which do not allow the formation of $\propto$ helix: Proline and hydroxyprolinc
30. Most stable protein structure is: Right handed alpha helix.
31. Amino acid sequence of protein can be determined by: Edman's method , Sanger's method (1 – Fluoro 2, 4,-dinitrobenzene).
32. Secondary and tertiary structure is determined by: X – ray crystallography, optical rotatory dispersion, nuclear magnetic resonance.
33. The structure of protein that is not disrupted by denaturation is: Primary structure.
34. Denaturing agents disrupt the peptide structure by breaking: Hydrogen bond.
35. The most rigid bond is between:'C' and 'N – atom(peptide bond).

Metabolism of Amino Acids

A. Catabolism of amino nitrogen of amino acids

1. The susceptibility of protein to degradation is expressed as: Half life of a protein.
2. The primary means by which amino acid derived nitrogen is metabolized is by the sequential action of: Aminotransferases, glutamate dehydrogenase and the urea cycle.
3. The enzymes that degrade proteins are: Intracellular proteases and peptidases.
4. In a normal adult , daily protein turnover per day is: 1 – 2%.
5. All amino acids undergo transamination reaction except: Lysine, threonine, proline, hydroxyproline.
6. Important transaminases of body are: Aspartate transaminase and alanine transaminase.
7. Amino acid released by breakdown of tissue proteins are used for:
   1. New protein synthesis
   2. Synthesis of non protein nitrogenous compounds
   3. Degraded
8. Biosynthesis of urea is divided into 4 stages:
   (i) Transamination
   (ii) Oxidative deamination
   (iii) Ammonia Transport
   (iv) Reactions of urea cycle.
9. The only amino acid in humans that can undergo oxidative deamination is: L – Glutamate.
10. Glutamine serves as a means of ammonia detoxification in: Kidney, CNS.
11. Another name of urea cycle: Krebs – Henselit cycle.
12. Rate limiting enzyme in urea synthesis is: Carbamoyl phosphate synthase I.
13. Normal plasma urea level is: 20 – 40 mg/dl.

B. Synthesis of nonessential amino acids and catabolism of carbon skeleton of amino acids

1. Important proteolytic enzymes of the body are: Pepsin, trypsin, chymotrypsim carboxypeptidase A and B and elastase.
2. A condition resulting from premature activation of the trypsinogen inside the pancreas itself is: Acute pancreatitis.
3. Absorption of neutral amino acids in renal tubules and brain is by the: Gamma glutamyl cycle.
4. Cathepsins are enzymes found in: Phagolysosomes.
5. Glutamic acid is synthesized from: ∝–Ketoglutarate.
6. Glutamine is synthesised from: Glutamic acid.
7. Glutamate is an important: Excitatory neurotransmitter.
8. Important metabolic role of glutamine is: Source of N atoms for the synthesis of purines and pyrimidines
9. The malate aspartate shuttle is important for: Transferring the cytoplasmic NADH into

mitochondria for oxidation in the ETC.

10. L – asparaginase is: Anticancer drug against leukemias and lymphomas.
11. Chief glucogenic amino acid: Alanine.
12. Carnosine is a dipeptide of: Histidine and β alanine.
13. β–alanine is used for the synthesis of: Coenzyme A.
14. Glycine may be used for the biosynthesis of:
    (i) Heme
    (ii) Creatine
    (iii) Purine nucleotides
    (iv) Glutathione
15. Immediate source of energy in muscles is: Creatine phosphate.
16. Oxalate renal stones are precipitated by the urinary excretion of amino acid: Glycine.
17. Uses of serine analogues:
    (i) Azaserine – Anticancer drug.
    (ii) Cycloserine - Antituberculous drug.
18. A site for phosphorylation in protein is: -OH groups of threonine residues.
19. The initiating amino acid in the synthesis of polypepetide chain in humans is: Methionine.
20. Cysteine is formed from: Serine and methionine.
21. Taurine, required for conjugation of bile acids is synthesised from: Cysteine.
22. Cystinuria is attributed to: The deficiency in transport of amino acids.
23. Amino acids excreted in cystinuria: Cystine, lysine, arginine, ornithine.
24. The risk of coronary artery disease is increased by increase in the levels of amino acid: Homocysteine.
25. Bacterial putrefaction of lysine in the intestine gives rise to: Cadaverine.
26. Highly basic amino acid is: Arginine.
27. Arginine is the precursor of: Nitric oxide.
28. Polyamines are: Spermine, spermidine and putrescine.
29. Branched chain amino acids are: Valine, leucine, isoleucine.
30. The only amino acid which is only ketogenic is: Leucine.
31. Branched chain amino acids undergo transamination to produce: Branched chain α-keto acid.
32. Deficiency of vitamin B_{12} impairs the metabolisms of: Valine, methyl malonyl CoA.
33. Cheesy odour of breath is seen in: Isovaleric acidemia.
34. The enzyme involved in hydroxylation of phenylalanine to tyrosine is: Phenylanine hydroxylase.
35. A drug in parkinsonism is: L – Dopa.
36. Catabolic product of adrenaline is: Vanillyl mandelic acid (VMA).

37. In alkaptonuria ochronosis occurs due to formation of: Polymer of benzoquinone acetate.
38. Cabbage like odour is found in: Acute tyrosinosis.
39. If urine sample darkens on standing, the most likely condition is: Alkaptonuria.
40. Tryptophan is oxidised by enzyme: Tryptophan pyrolase.
41. Kynureninase enzyme of tryptophan catabolism is dependent on: Pyridoxal phosphate.
42. About 60 mg of tryptophan is equivalent to: 1 mg of nicotinic acid.
43. Degradation product of histidine metabolism: Urocanate.
44. Enzyme deficiency found in histidinemia is: Histidase.
45. Oral challenge with histidine in folate deficiency increases the excretion of: Formiminoglutamate in urine.

TABLE 1: Amino acid requirements of humans

Nutritionally essentials	Non essential	Semi essential
Valine	Alanine	Arginine
Leucine	Aspartate	Histidine
Isoleucine	Asparagine	
Lysine	Glutamate	
Methionine	Glutamine	
Phenyl alanine	Glycine	
Tryptophan	Serine	
Threonine	Cysteine, Proline, Hydroxy-proline, Hydroxylysine, Tyrosine	

TABLE 2

	Non essential amino acid	Precursor compound
1	Glycine	Serine, Choline, Glyoxylate
2	Alanine	Pyruvate
3	Serine	3 – phosphoglycerate, Glycine
4	Glutamic acid	α-Ketoglutarate
5	Glutamine	Glutamic acid
6	Aspartic acid	Oxaloacetate
7	Asparagine	Aspartic acid
8	Tyrosine	Phenyl alanine
9	Cysteine	Homocysteine, serine
10	Proline	Glutamate
11	Hydroxy proline	Proline
12	Hydroxy lysine	Lysine

TABLE 3: Amino acidurias

Disorder	Abnormality or absence of	Clinical manifestation	Substance in blood	Substance in urine	Treatment
Phenyl ketonuria (PKU) Type I classical	Phenyl alanine-hydroxylase	MR, hypertonia, seizure	Phenyl alanine	Phenyl pyruvate	Dietary restriction of Phenylalamine
Type II	PAH deficiency	Mild MR	Phe	Phenyl pyruvate	do
Type IV	Dihydropterin deficiency	Neurological	Phe	--	DOPA 5-OH-tryptophan
Hpertyrosinemia	Fumarylace-toacetate hydrolase	MR, hepatorenal damage	Tyrosine, Methionine	Tyrosine, PHPPA	Restrict Phe and Tyr
Tyrosinemia Type II	Tyrosine amino trasferase	MR eye, skin	Tyrosine	Tyrosine, Tyramine	Do
Alkaptonuria	Homogentisic acid oxidase	Arthritis, cartilage pigments	Homogentisic acid	Homogentisic acid	Nil
Homocystinuria (Type 1)	Cystathionine beta synthase	MR, Ectopia lentis, seizures	Homocysteine, Methionine	Homocystine	Cysteine ↑ methionine ↓ Folate
Homocystinura (Type 2)	Methyl trans-ferase	MR	Homocysteine	Homocystine	Folate
Homocystinura (type 3)	Methylene THFA reductase	MR	Homocysteine	Homocystine	Restrict Histidine
Histidinemia	Histidase	MR, speech defect	Histidine, alanine	Imidazol pyruvic acid	Restrict Histidine
Maple syrup urine disease	Branched chain keto acid decarboxylase	Maple syrup odour acidosis	Val, Leu,Ile, keto acids	Val, Leu,Ile, keto acids	Ristrict Val, leu, Ile.
Hyperglycinemia	Glycine cleavage system	MR, seizures	Glycine spasticity	Glycine	None
Propionic acidemia	Propionyl CoA carboxylase	MR seizures ketosis	Propionate	Propionate	Low protein diet
Methyl malonic aciduria	Methyl malonyl CoA mutase	MR, ketosis hypotonia	Methyl matonic acid	Methyl malonic acid; ketonebodies	Vitamin B12
Cystathionuria	Cystathionase	Benign	Cystathionine	Cystathionine	None required
Carnosinemia	Carnosinase	Neurological	Carnosine	Carnosine	Nil
Hyperprolinemia	Proline oxidase	Benign	Proline	Proline hydroxyproline	--
Citrullinemia	Arginino succi-nate synthetase	MR seizures vommiting	Ammonia, citrulline	Citrulline	Low protein; high Arg
Artgininmia	Arginase	Spastic diplegia vomit	Arginine ammonia	Arginine, ornithine	Low protein diet
Hyperornit-hinemia	Ornithine decarboxylase	Vomiting lethergy	Ornithine; ammonia	Ornithine	do
OTC deficiency	Ornithine transcarbamoy-lase	Lethargy convulsions	Ammonia	Orotic acid; uracil; glutamine	do
CPSI deficiency	Carbamoyl phosphate synthetase I	Vomiting lethargy	Ammonia glutamine	Glutamine	do
Argininosuccinic aciduria	Argininosuccinate lyase	Vomiting trichortia nodose	Arginino-succinate, citrulline	Argininosuc-cinate; citrulline	Arginine ↑ Protein ↓

TABLE 4: Amino acid derived compounds of Biologic importance

Compound	Precursor Amino acid	Primary Function
1. Creatine Phosphate	Glycine, Arginine	Energy storage compound
2. Carnitine	Lysine	Fatty acid transporter
3. Dopamine	Tyrosine	Neurotransmitter
4. Epinephrine	Tyrosine, Methionine	Hormone
5. Norepinephrine	Tyrosine	Neurotransmitter
6. Thyroxine	Tyrosine	Hormone
7. Melanin	Tyrosine	Colour pigment
8. Melatonin	Tryptophan	Hormone
9. GABA	Glutamate	Neurotransmitter
10. Serotonin	Tryptophan	Vasoconstrictor
11. Histamine	Histidine	Vasodilator
12. Nitric oxide	Arginine	Vasodilator, Neurotransmitter
13. Polyamines	Ornithine, Methionine	Cell proliferation, synthesis of DNA and RNA, protein biosynthesis
14 Sphingosine	Serine	Alcohol of Sphingolipids

SOLVED QUESTIONS

Q.1. Structural proteins are: **(AIPGME 1994)**

1. Fibrous

2. Globular

3. Branched

4. Compound.

Ans. **1**

Structural proteins are collagen, elastin, keratins. Collagen is the most abundant protein in mammals and is the main fibrous component of skin, bone, tendon, cartilage and teeth. Fibrous proteins have axial ratio of 10 or more.

Q.2. The tertiary structure of protein is most commonly detected by: **(AIPG 1994)**

1. X-ray crystallography

2. Spectrophotometry

3. Electrophoresis

4. Chromatography.

Ans. **1**

The secondary and tertiary structure of protein is determined by X-ray crystallography. The three dimensional structure of thousand of proteins have been determined by x-ray crystallography. In X-ray crystallography, a beam of X-ray is diffracted by the electrons around each atom and the intensity of diffracted beam is detected by a photographic plate. Electrophoresis and chromatography techniques are useful for isolation of individual amino acids or proteins from a mixture. Spectrophotometry is used for enzymatic activity studies.

Q.3. Flexibility of protein depends on: (AIPGME 1994)

1. **Glycine**
2. **Tryptophan**
3. **Phenyl alanine**
4. **Histidine**

Ans. **1**

Glycine is seen where the polypeptide chain bends or turns. Glycine has a small size and also does not cause a steric hindrance so is responsible for flexibility of protein.

Q.4. Amino acid which lacks chirality is: (AIPGME 1996)

1. **Lysine**
2. **Leucine**
3. **Histidine**
4. **Glycine.**

Ans. **4**

The carbon atom attached to four different atoms or groups of atom is called a chiral carbon atom. Amino acids possessing chiral carbon atom in their structure possess optical activity (chirality). Glycine is the simplest amino acid and has no asymmetric carbon atom and therefore shows no optical activity.

COOH
|
H—C—NH_2
|
H Glycine

Q.5. An amino acid which does not participate by α-helix formation is: (AIPGME 1996)

1. **Leucine**
2. **Glycine**
3. **Proline**
4. **Lysine.**

Ans. **3**

The alpha helix is a spiral structure. The polypeptide bonds form the back bone and the side chains of amino acids extend outward. The structure is stabilized by hydrogen bonds between NH_2 group of fourth amino acid and C=0 of first amino acid. Proline is an imino acid (no free $-NH_2$ group N) so proline can not form the correct pattern of hydrogen bonds. It is found at the end of the α -helix where it alters the direction of the polypeptide chain and terminates the helix.

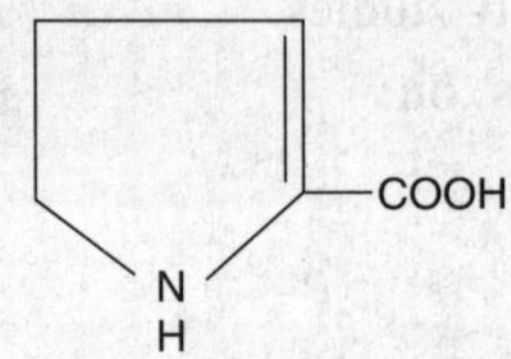

Q.6. Transamination of pyruvate and glutamic acid leads to the formation of: **(AIPGME 1996)**

1. **Oxaloacetate**
2. **α-ketoglutarate**
3. **Aspartate**
4. **Malate.**

Ans. **2**

Transamination is the exchange of the α-amino group between one α- amino acid and another α-ketoacid forming a new pair of α-amino acid and α-keto acid.

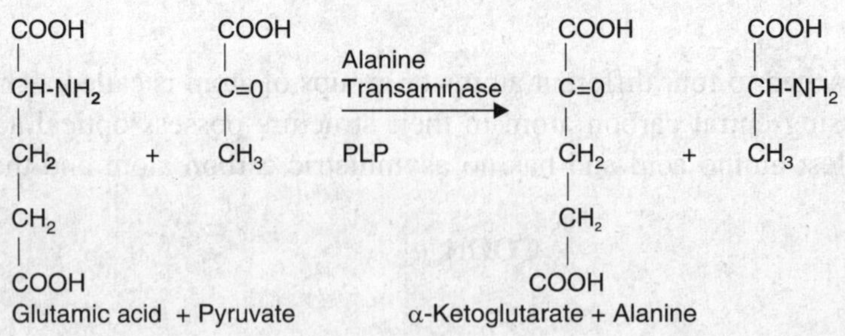

Q.7. Which of the following is a denaturing substance? **(AIPGME 1996)**

1. **Guanosine**
2. **Guanidine**
3. **Glutamate**
4. **Glycine.**

Ans. **2**

Non covalent interactions in a protein may be disrupted by guanidine hydrochloride. This leads to separation of polypeptide chains. Gluamate and glycine are amino acids. Guanosine is a nucleoside.

Q.8. Property of photochromosity is seen amongst the following amino acids: (AIPGME 1997)

1. **Unsaturated amino acid**
2. **Aromatic amino acid**
3. **Monocarboxylic acid**
4. **dicarboxylic acid.**

Ans. 2

Q.9. Leucine is a amino acid with a: (AIPGME 1998)

1. **Nonpolar side chain**
2. **Polar side chain**
3. **Negatively charged side chain**
4. **Positively charged side chain.**

Ans. 1

Leucine

COOH These groups are hydrophobic and lipophilic

|

$CH-NH_2$

|

CH_2

|

$HC - CH_3$

|

CH_3

Q.10. Transamination of pyruvate with glutamate produces: (AIPGME 1998)

1. **Oxaloacetate and aspartate**
2. **Alanine and aspartate**
3. **Oxaloacetate and α-ketoglutarate**
4. **Alanine and α- ketoglutarate.**

Ans. 4

Explanation same as Q.6

Q.11. Most basic amino acid out of the following is: (AIPGME 1998)

1. **Alanine**
2. **Arginine**
3. **Histidine**
4. **Lysine.**

Ans. 2

There are two basic amino acids lysine and arginine. Out of these two most basic amino acid is arginine.

Arginine

COOH

$CHNH_2$

CH_2

CH_2

CH_2

NH

C = NH

NH_2

Lysine

COOH

$CH-NH_2$

CH_2

CH_2

CH_2

$CH_2—NH_2$

Q.12. Optically inactive amino acid is: **(AIPGME 1999)**

1. **Proline**
2. **Glycine**
3. **Lysine**
4. **Leucine.**

Ans. **2**

Explanation same as Q.4

Q.13. Most nonpolar amino acid is: **(AIPGME 2000)**

1. **Leucine**
2. **Glycine**
3. **Arginine**
4. **Lysine**

Ans. **1**

Side chain present in nonpolar amino acid is aliphatic or aromatic These groups are hydrophobic and lipophilic. Other nonpolar (hydrophobic) amino acids are alanine, isoleucine, methionine, proline, valine, phenylalanine and tryptophan.

Q.14. Basic amino acids are: **(AIPGME 2001)**

1. **Aspartate and glutamate**
2. **Serine and glycine**
3. **Lysine and arginine**
4. **None of the above**

Ans. **3**

Explanation same as Q.11

Q.15. Amino acid with dissociation constant closest to physiological pH is:

1. **Serine**
2. **Histidine**
3. **Threonine**
4. **Proline.**

Ans. 2

At dissociation constant (pk) point 50% molecules are in cation or in anion form depending on pH while rest 50% molecules are in zwitter ions form. The buffering action is maximum in and around dissociation constant and minimum at isoelectric pH. The pk value of imidazolium group of histidine is 6.1 and therefore effective as a buffer at the physiological pH of 7.4

Q.16. Elasticity of the corneal layer of skin is due to the presence of:

1. **Histidine**
2. **Keratine**
3. **Lysine**
4. **Cysteine.**

Ans. 2

Q.17. The primary role of chaperones is to help in: (AIPGME 2003)

1. **Protein synthesis**
2. **Protein degradation**
3. **Protein denaturation**
4. **Protein folding.**

Ans. 4

Chaperone proteins participate in the folding of over half of mammalian proteins. The central cavity of hsp 60 (60 – κ Da heat shock protein) chaperone provides a sheltered environment in which a polypeptide can fold until all hydrophobic regions are buried in its interior, eliminating aggregation.

Q.18. Which of the following group of proteins assist in the 'folding' of other proteins?:

1. **Proteases**
2. **Proteosomes**
3. **Templates**
4. **Chaperones.**

Ans. 4

[Explanation same as Q. 17]

Q.19. Cytochrome C of the bacteria has 50% identity of amino acid sequence with that of human. Which of the following is the most conserved parameter in these two proteins? (AIPGME 2004)

1. **Quaternary structure**

2. **Tertiary structure**
3. **Amino acid sequence**
4. **Loop and turn segments**

Ans. 2

Q.20. Alpha helix and Beta pleated sheet are examples of: **(AIPGME 2004)**

1. **Primary structure**
2. **Secondary structure**
3. **Tertiary structure**
4. **Quaternary structure.**

Ans. 2

Both α-helix and β-pleated sheet are examples of secondary structure of protein. The linear sequene of amino acid (primary structure) is folded spirally to form α- helix or two linear chains of polypeptide lie near to each other either in parallel or in antiparallel direction.

Q.21. The amino acid residue having an imino side chain is: **(AIPGME 2005)**

1. **Lysine**
2. **Histidine**
3. **Tyrosine**
4. **Proline.**

Ans. 4

Proline and hydroxyproline are imino acids

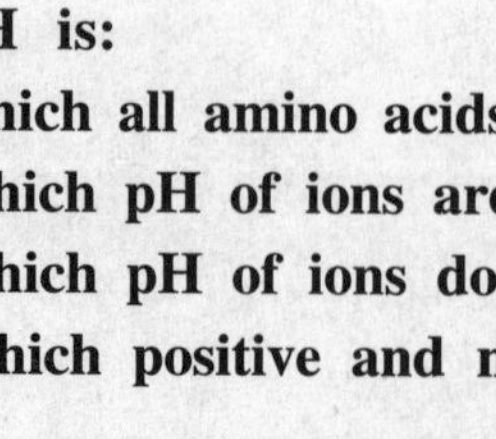

Proline

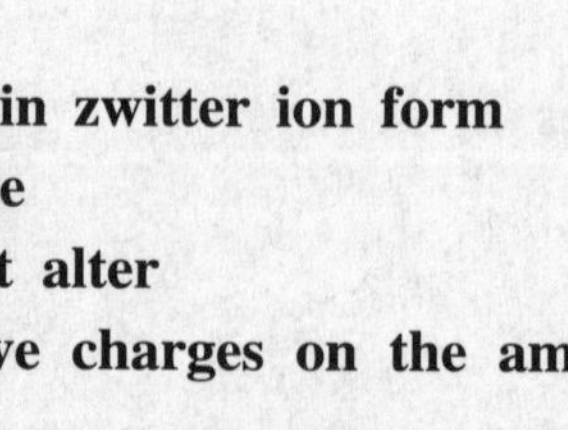

Hydroxy proline

Q.22. Isoselectric pH is: **(AIIMS JUNE 1998)**

1. **Point at which all amino acids are in zwitter ion form**
2. **Point at which pH of ions are same**
3. **Point at which pH of ions does not alter**
4. **Point at which positive and negative charges on the aminoacid are equal.**

Ans. 4

The pH at which the molecules carries no net charge is known as isoelectric pH All the groups are ionized but positive and negative charges are equal so the charges will cancel each other. At isoelectric pH amino acid exists in a zwitter ion form.

Q.23. Sequence in a long chain of protein is identified by:

1. **Restriction fragment length polymorphism (RFLP)**
2. **Chromosome walking**
3. **Leucine zipper**
4. **SSOP.**

Ans. 2

Chromosome walking studies are used to find out DNA sequence. From DNA sequence, sequence in a long chain of proteins can also be determined.

Q.24. The property of proteins to absorb ultraviolet rays of light is due to:

1. **Peptide bond**
2. **Imino group**
3. **Disulphide bond**
4. **Aromatic amino acid.**

Ans. 4

Q.25. Which of these amino acids will migrate slowest to the anode end at the physiological pH: **(AIIMS May 2001)**

1. **Aspartic acid**
2. **Glycine**
3. **Lysine**
4. **Valine.**

Ans. 3

Acidic amino acids are aspartic acid and glutamic acid. They have two-COOH groups and one – NH_2 group. At physiological pH, their side chains are ionized having a –COO-group.

Basic amino acids are arginine, lysine and histidine. They have two – NH_2 groups and one – COOH group. At physiological pH, they have ionised – NH_3^+ group.

So at the physiological pH, amino acid carrying positive charge will move slowest to the anode. Glycine and valine are neutral amino acids.

Q.26. Most stable amino acid at the physiological pH is: **(AIIMS May 2001)**

1. **Histidine**
2. **Lysine**
3. **Arginine**
4. **Glycine.**

Ans. 1

The dissociation constant (pk) of imidazolium group of histidine is 6.1 which is close to physiological pH (7.4) so at physiological pH, histidine has buffering capacity so it is not converted to “zwitter ion” form.

Q.27. Which of these amino acids does not have anomeric carbon atom:

(AIIMS May 2002)

1. **Valine**
2. **Alanine**
3. **Tyrosine**
4. **Glycine.**

Ans. 4

Explanation same as Q.4

Q.28. Defect in folding of the protein result in which of the following clinical disease:

1. **Kuru**
2. **Migraine**
3. **Hypothyroidism**
4. **Myopia.**

Ans. 1

Q.29. An alfa helix of a protein is most likely to be disrupted if a missense mutation introduces the following amino acid within the alpha helical structure:

(AIIMS Nov 2002)

1. **Alanine**
2. **Aspartic acid**
3. **Tyrosin**
4. **Glycine.**

Ans. 4

Q.30. The primary structure of a protein refers to: **(AIIMS May 2004)**

1. **Linear structure and order of the amino acids present**
2. **Regular confirmational forms of a protein**
3. **Complete three-dimensional structure of the polypeptide units of a given protein**
4. **Subunit structure of the protein.**

Ans. 1

Primarry structure is the linear sequence of amino acids held together by peptide bonds in its peptide chain. The primary structure of a protein is largely responsible for its function.

Q.31. Which one of the following is not true for an α- helix: **(AIIMS May 2004)**

1. **It is one of the most important secondary structure**
2. **It has a net dipole moment**
3. **All hydrogen bonds are aligned in the same direction**

4. Long stretches of left handed α-helix occur in proteins.

Ans. **4**

α-Helix and β-pleated sheet are the two types of secondary structures. In α-helix intra chain hydrogen bonding is present. Hydrogen bond is present between carbonyl oxygen of 1st amino acid and amide nitrogen of fourth amino acid residues. Thus they are aligned in the same direction.

Left handed α -helix is less stable than right handed α-helix because of the steric interference between the C=O and the side chains. Only the right handed α-helix has been found in protein structure.

Q.32. The molecular weight of a protein can be determined by: (AIIMS Nov 2005)

1. Native poly acrylamide gel electrophoresis (PAGE)

2. Sodium dodecyl sulphate SDS-PAGE

3. Isoelectric focussing

4. Ion exchange chromatography.

Ans. **2**

The proteins in general have a large molecular weight. Molecular weight is determined by physical methods such as osmotic pressure measurement, depression in freezing point, light scattering effect, 'x'-ray diffraction, turbidity measurement and now a days by specialised methods such as analytical ultracentrifugation, molecular sieving by gel filtration and sodium dodecyl sulphate (SDS) - polyacrylamide gel electrophoresis.

Q.33. If chymotrypsin molecule undergoes a ser - 195 - ala mutation then: (AIPGME 1998)

1. Chymotrypsin will not bind the substrate

2. Chymotrypsin will bind the substrate as well as cause cleavage

3. Chymotrypsin will bind the substrate but will not cause cleavage

4. No effect will be observed.

Ans. **3**

In the activation of chymotrypsinogen to chymotrypsin , trypsin will act on it in such a manner that A peptide (1-13 amino acids), B peptide (16-46) and C peptide (149-245) are formed. These 3 segments are approximated, so that the active sites contain histidine (57) and aspartic acid (102) residues of β peptide and serine (195) on C peptide. Replacement of serine (195) by alanine changes polar amino acid by nonpolar residue. So the enzyme will bind with the substrate but does not bring out its cleavage.

Q.34. True statement regarding Nitric oxide is: (AIPGME 1999)

1. NO is synthesised from arginine

2. NO is spontaneously produced from NO_2

3. NO causes vasoconstriction

4. NO is released from mitochondria

Ans. 1

Nitric oxide is formed from arginine by the enzyme nitric oxide synthase .The guanidino nitrogen of arginine is incorporated into NO. From the molecular oxygen, one atom is incorporated to NO and the other into citrulline.

Metabolic fate of NO involves its combination with oxygen to form NO_2. These nitrites are excreted through urine. Nitric oxide is a potent vasodilator.

There are 3 isoforms of nitric oxide synthase (NOS) – Neuronal NOS , inducible (macrophage) NOS and endothelial NOS.

Q.35. Which of the following amino acid is excreted in urine inmaple syrup urine disease: (AIPGME 1999)

1. **Tryptophan**
2. **Phenylalanine**
3. **Leucine**
4. **Arginine.**

Ans. 3

Maple syrup urine disease is a inherited disorder of branched chain amino acids (Valine, leucine and isoleucine). The basic biochemical defect is deficient carboxylation of branched chain keto acids produced from these amino acids. So there is excretion of branched chain keto acids and amino acids.

Q.36. Ammonia is detoxified in brain to: (AIPGME 1999)

1. **Urea**
2. **Glutamine**
3. **GABA**
4. **Uric acid.**

Ans. 2

Being highly toxic, ammonia should be eliminated or detoxified as and when it is formed. Even very minute quantity of ammonia may produce toxicity in central nervous system. In brain cells, the intracellular ammonia is trapped by glutamic acid to form glutamine.

Q.37. Mechanism of action of nitric oxide is through: (AIPGME 2001)

1. **cGMP**
2. **cAMP**
3. **Ca^{++}**
4. **Tyrosine.**

Ans. 1

Nitric oxide activates guanylate cyclase which causes formation of cGMP. Vasodilation effect of nitric oxide and inhibition of platelet aggregation are mediated through cGMP and protein kinase .

Q.38. Source of the nitrogen in urea cycle are: (AIPGME 2001)

1. **Aspartate and ammonia**
2. **Glutamate and ammonia**
3. **Arginine and ammonia**
4. **Uric acids.**

Ans. 1

The two nitrogen atoms of urea are derived from two different sources, one from ammonia and the other directly from the alpha amino group of aspartic acid.

Q.39. If urine sample darkens on standing: the most likely condition is: (AIPGME 2001)

1. **Phenyl ketonuria**
2. **Alkaptonuria**
3. **Maple syrup disease**
4. **Tyrosinemia.**

Ans. 2

Alkaptonuria is an autosomal recessive disease due to deficiency of homogentisate oxidase. Homogentisic acid is produced during tyrosine metabolism.

$$\text{Pnenyl alanine} \longrightarrow \text{Tyrosine} \longrightarrow \text{Homogentisic acid} \xrightarrow[\text{oxidase}]{\text{Homogentisate}} \text{Fumarate}$$

Deficiency of homogentisate oxidase causes accumulation of homogentisic acid which is oxidised and polymerized to black coloured alkaptone bodies.These gets deposited at various sites causing ochronosis. Thus urine turns black on standing because of oxidation of homogentisate.

Q.40. A baby presents with refusal to feed, skin lesions, seizures, ketosis, organic acid in urine with normal ammonia; likely diagnosis is: (AIPGME 2001)

1. **Propionic aciduria**
2. **Multiple carboxylase deficiency**
3. **Maple syrup urine disease**
4. **Urea cycle enzyme deficiency.**

Ans. 2

Q.41. Nitric oxide synthase: (AIPGME 2002)

1. **Is inhibited by Ca^{++}**
2. **Catalyzes a dioxygenase reaction**
3. **Accepts electrons from NADH**
4. **Requires NADPH, FAD, FMN and heme iron.**

Ans. 4

Nitric oxide synthase is a dimeric protein. It contains heme, FAD , FMN, tetrahydro biopterine and calmodulin. The enzyme utilizes NADPH and molecular oxygen. The guanidino nitrogen of arginine is incorporated into nitric oxide. From the molecular oxygen, one atom is added to NO and the other into citrulline.

Q.42. Phenylalanine is the precursor of all of the following except: (AIPGME 2002)

1. **Tyrosine**
2. **Epinephrine**
3. **Thyroxine**
4. **Melatonin.**

Ans. 4

Tyrosine is a nonessential amino acid formed from phenylalanine. Tyrosine is a precursor of epinephrine,norepinephrine, tri-iodo thyronine and thyroxine.Melatonin is formed form tryptophan. Tryptophan is first converted to serotonin which is then converted to melatonin.

Q.43. A child presents with metabolic lactic acidosis along with hyperammonemia and convulsion is due to: (AIIMS June 2000)

1. **Reye's syndrome**
2. **Mitochondrial enzyme disorders (MELAS)**
3. **Urea cycle defect**
4. **Phenylketonuria.**

Ans. 1

In urea cycle only hyperammonia is seen; no lactic acidosis, no convulsion. In phenylketonuria, there is no lactic acidosis .Thus, the above mentioned condition is neither of urea cycle defect nor of phenylketonuria. Both Reye's syndrome and mitochondrial enzyme disorders (MELAS) are mitochondrial encephalopathies. Seizures, hyperammonemia and lactic acidosis are seen in Reye's syndrome while in MELAS only lactic acidosis is seen and there is no hyperammonemia. But recurrent episodes of strokes are the main clinical feature in MELAS.

Q.44. Increased risk of myocardial infarction is associated with which amino acid: (AIIMS May 2001)

1. **Methionine**
2. **Homocystine**
3. **Ornithine**
4. **Valine.**

Ans. 2

Excess homocysteine interact with lysyl residues of collagen forming homocysteine thiolactone which thiolates free - NH_2 groups in LDL and causes, them to aggregate and be endocytosed by macrophages. The lipid content of LDL deposits forming atheromas. Other effect of homocysteine are lipid peroxidation and platelet aggregation which leads to fibrosis and calcification of atherosclerotic plaque .

An increase of 5 μmol /L of homocysteine in serum elevates the risk of coronary artery disease by as much as cholesterol increase of 20 mg/dl.

Q.45. Which end product of citric acid cycle is used in detoxification of ammonia in brain: (AIIMS May 2001)

1. **Oxaloacetate**
2. **Alpha ketoglutarate**
3. **Succinate**
4. **Citrate.**

Ans. 2

Alpha ketoglutaric acid is one of the intrmediate of citric acid cycle. It is converted to glutamic acid This glutamic acid in brain cells accept NH_3 and forms glutamine which is the transport form of ammonia from brain.

Q.46. Amino acids secreted in cystinuria are all except: (AIIMS May 2001)

1. **Ornithine**
2. **Histidine**
3. **Arginine**
4. **Lysine.**

Ans. 2

In cystinuria there is excretion of cystine, ornithine, lysine and arginine. The disorder is due to the deficiency in transport of amino acids.

Q.47. Which of the following groups of proteins assist in the folding of other proteins:

1. **Proteases**
2. **Proteosomes**
3. **Templates**
4. **Chaperones.**

Ans. 4

Explanation same as Q.17

Q.48. Melanin pigment formed from:

1. **Tryptophan**
2. **Arginine**
3. **Phenyl alanine**
4. **Valine.**

Ans. 3

Phenylalanine is converted to tyrosine which is then metabolized to give various important substances. These include melanin, catecholamines and thyroid hormones.

Q.49. The reducing end of glutathione , the amino acid is:

1. **Glycine**
2. **Leucine**
3. **Cysteine**
4. **Valine.**

Ans. 3

Glutathione is gamma glutamyl cysteinyl glycine . It is abbreviated as GSH , to indicate the reactive -SH group. Role of glutathione is mainly in reduction reactions because of -SH group of cysteine.

Q.50. Amino acid which functions as a free radical scavenger is:

1. **Glycine**
2. **Cystine**
3. **Cysteine**
4. **Glutamine.**

Ans. 3

The cysteine is derived from glutathione, which is the active conjugating agent. –SH group of cysteine from glutathione donates H^+ ion to detoxify the peroxides and free radicals formed.

Q.51. Following are the essential amino acids:

1. **Phenylalanine, Tryptophan, Lysine**
2. **Phenylalanine, Arginine, Methionine**
3. **Phenylalanine, Valine, Glycine**
4. **Histidine, Glutamine, Valine**

Ans. 1

Essential amino acids are not synthesised in the body so they are supplied in food for normal growth. The essential amino acids include-isoleucine, leucine,threonine, lysine, methionine, phenylalanine, tryptophan and valine. Arginine and histidine are semiessential amino acids while rest all are non essential amino acids.

Q.52. Cytochromes are:

1. **Pyridine nucleotides**
2. **Riboflavin containing nucleotides**
3. **Metal containing flavoproteins**
4. **Iron-porphyrin proteins.**

Ans. 4

Cytochromes (Fe and Cu) and chlorophyll (Mg) are the proteins that contains metal containing tetrapyrrole prosthetic groups.

Q.53. Ammonia is detoxified in liver to form:

1. **Uric acid**

2. **Glutamine**
3. **Creatinine**
4. **Urea.**

Ans. 4

Ammonia is highly toxic. So in vertebrates it is converted to urea in liver. Hepatic urea synthesis takes place in part in the mitochondrial matrix and in part in the cytosol.

Q.54. In Hartnup's disease... is excreated in the urine:

1. **Ornithine**
2. **Glutamine**
3. **Tryptophan**
4. **Phenylalanine.**

Ans. 3

During Hartnup's disease indole derivatives of unabsorbed tryptophan formed by intestinal bacteria is excreted in the urine.

Q.55. Guanido acetate is converted to:

1. **Creatinine**
2. **Creatine phosphate**
3. **Choline**
4. **Hydroxyproline.**

Ans. 2

Guanidoacetate (Glycocyamine) is converted to creatin phosphate during the biosynthesis and metabolism of creatine and creatinine.

Q.56. Which of the following is a precursor of protoporphyrin:

1. **Alanine**
2. **Leucine**
3. **Histidine**
4. **Glycine.**

Ans. 4

The product of the condensation reaction between succinyl COA and glycine is α-amino β-ketoadipic acid, which is rapidly decarboxylated to form α-amino levulinate (ALA) via ALA synthase, which is the rate limiting enzyme in porphyrin biosynthesis.

Q.57. Alkaptonuria is due to the defective amino acid metabolism of:

1. **Tyrosine**
2. **Tryptophan**
3. **Leucine**
4. **Isoleucine**

Ans. 1

Alkaptonuria is caused due to the deficiency of enzyme homogentisate oxidase during tyrosine metabolism. During this the urine darkens on exposure to air due to oxidation of excreted homogentisate. Late in the disease, there is arthritis and connective tissue pigmentation due to oxidation of homogentisate to benzoquinone acetate, which polymerizes and binds to connective tissue.

Q.58. Melanin is synthesized from:

1. **Glycine**
2. **Leucine**
3. **Threonine**
4. **Phenylalanine.**

Ans. 4

Melanine is a metabolite formed during the metabolism of phenylalaine is converted to tyrosine which is then give rise to melanin.

Q.59. Serotonin is derived from:

1. **Phenylalanine**
2. **Serine**
3. **Tryptophan**
4. **Cysteine.**

Ans. 3

Hydroxylation of tryptophan to 5-hydroxy tryptophan by liver tyrosine hydroxylase. Subsequent decarboxylation forms serotonin (5-hydroxytryptoamine)

Q.60. Major source of ammonia in the kidney is:

1. **Urea**
2. **Aspartate**
3. **Glutamine**
4. **Glutamate.**

Ans. 3

Free ammonium ions and glutamine are formed by the interconversion from glutamate by glutamine synthase and glutaminase.

Q.61. All of the following are acute phase proteins except:

1. **Alpha-1 antitrypsin**
2. **Fibrinogen**
3. **Haptoglobin**
4. **Major basic protein.**

Ans. 4

The acute phase proteins are also known as reactants and includes C-reactive proteins, α_1-antitrypsin, haptoglobin, α_1-acid glycoproteins and fibrinogen.

Q.62. At physiological Ph, the carboxy terminal of a peptide is: (AIIMS Nov 2005)

1. **Positively charged.**
2. **Negatively charged.**
3. **Neutral.**
4. **Infinitely charged.**

Ans. 2

At physiological pH, the carboxy terminal of the peptide is negatively charged. As at physiological pH, the amino acids have both the negatively charged carboxyl ion ($-COO^-$) and the positively charged ammonium ion ($-NH_3^+$). Therefore, amino acids are also called as dipolar ion or zwitter ion.

Q.63. Substitution of which one of the following amino acids in place of alanine would increase the absorbance of protein at 280 nm: (AIIMS Nov 2005)

1. **Lucien.**
2. **Arginine.**
3. **Tryptophan.**
4. **Prolein.**

Ans. 3

Substitution of tryptophan in place of alanine would increase the absorbance of protein at 280 nm. This is because the tryptophan, tyrosine and phenylalanine are the only amino acids that can absorb ultraviolet light at 280 nm. Whereas the other amino acids do not absorb visible light hence they are colorless.

Q.64. Secretory proteins are synthesized in: (AIIMS Nov 2005)

1. **Cytoplasm.**
2. **Endoplasmic reticulum.**
3. **First in cytoplasm and then in endoplasmic reticulum.**
4. **First in endoplasmic reticulum and then in cytoplasm.**

Ans. 2

All type of protein synthesis takes place in ribosomes. But secretory proteins are synthesized in ribosomes attached to endoplasmic reticulum. As secretory proteins contain signal peptides, which help them to be transported into Golgi apparatus via endoplasmic reticulum where sorting of proteins for their respective destination occurs. Where as proteins which have to be delivered in the cytosol are synthesized in free ribosomes present in cytoplasm.

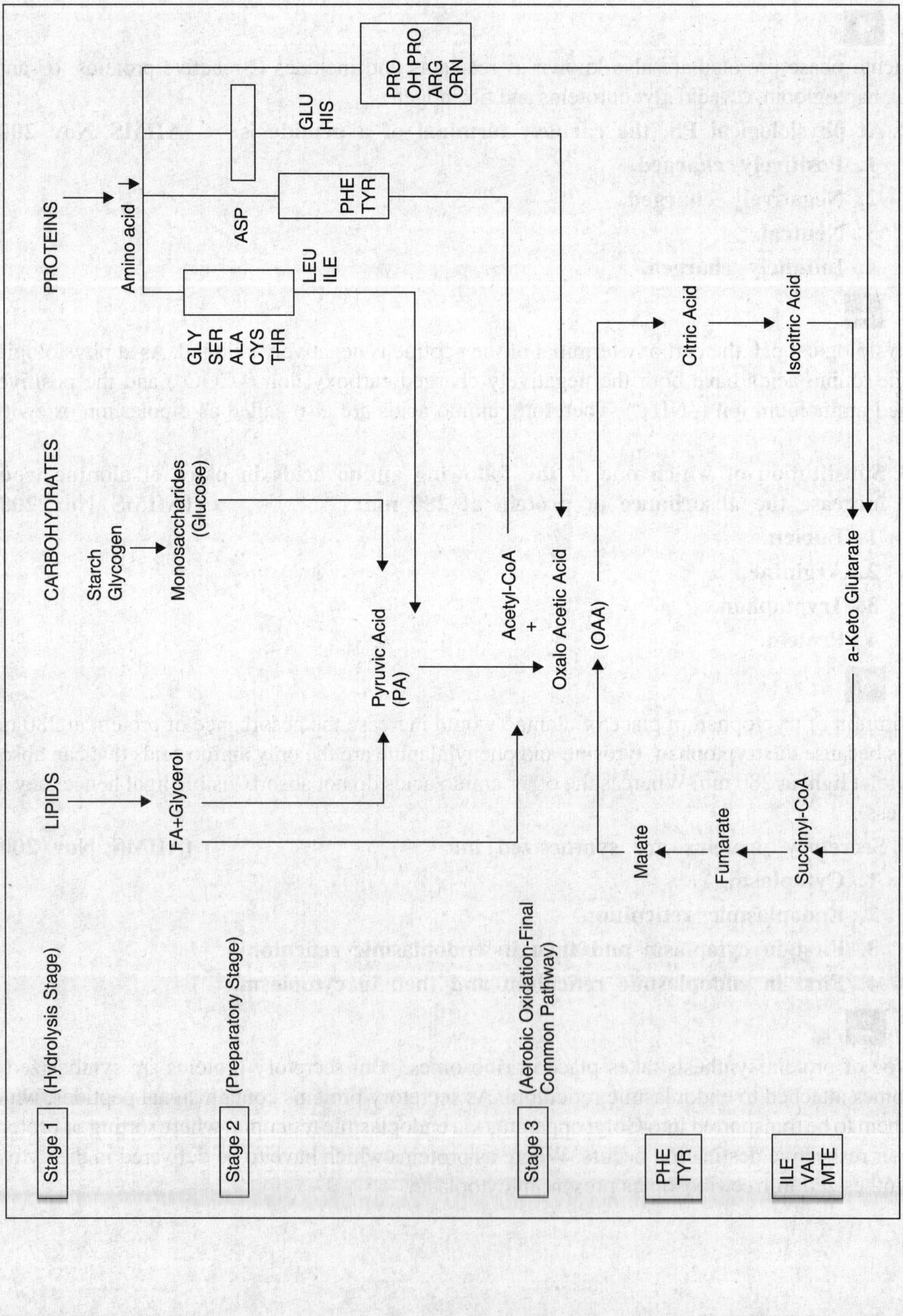

This figure shows the interrelationship between the three stages.

Q.65. If cellular proteins do not fold into a specific conformation, their functions are affected. Certain disorders arise, if specific proteins are misfolded. Which of the following disorders arises due to conformational isomerization: (AIIMS Nov 2005)

1. **Familial fatal insomnia.**
2. **Hepatitis delta.**
3. **Pernicious anemia.**
4. **Lesch-nyhan syndrome.**

Ans. 1

The conformational change in the protein structure leads to the loss of function of the protein. Some of the diseases that can be caused due to such type of alterations are:

Fatal familial insomnia and Creutzfeldt- Jacob's disease in humans.

Scrapie in sheep.

Bovine spongiform encephalopathy in cow etc.

Q.66. Which one of the following can be a homologous substitution for isoleucine in a protein sequence? (AIPGEE 2006)

1. **Methionine.**
2. **Aspartic acid.**
3. **Valine.**
4. **Arginine.**

Ans. 3

The best homologous substitution for isoleucine in a protein structure is valine. Because, valine, leucine and isoleucine are the branched chain and essential amino acid. These three amino acids initially undergo a common pathway and then diverge to result in different end products.

Q.67. Proteins are linear polymers of amino acids. They fold into compact structures. Sometimes, these folded structures associate to form homo or hetero dimers. Which one of the following refers to this associated form? (AIPGEE 2006)

1. **Denatured state.**
2. **Molecular aggregation.**
3. **Precipitation.**
4. **Quaternary structure.**

Ans. 4

Proteins are the polymers of L-α amino acids. The structure of the protein is rather complex which can be divided into four levels of organization-

1. Primary structure- The linear sequence of amino acid forming the backbone of proteins (polypeptides).
2. Secondary structure- The spatial arrangement of protein by twisting of the polypeptide chain.

3. Tertiary structure- it is the 3-D structure of the functional protein.
4. Quaternary structure- Some of the proteins are composed of two or more polypeptide chains reffered to as subunits. The spatial arrangements of these subunit is known as quaternary structure. Monomeric proteins consist of a single polypeptide chain. Dimeric proteins contain two-polypeptide chain, homodimers contain two copies of the same polypeptide chain, and while in a heterodimer the polypeptides differ. Greek letters are used to distinguish different subunits of heterooligomeric protein, and subscripts indicate the number of each subunit type. For example - a_4 designates a homotetrameric protein, and a_2b_2g a protein with five subunits of three different types.

Q.68. The comparison of the amino acid sequence of Cytochrome-C from different species shows many variations. Most of these variations are found: (AIPGEE 2006)

1. Randomly.
2. Only in helical regions.
3. Only in strand regions.
4. Mainly in loop regions.

Ans. 1

Most variations in amino acid sequence of Cytochrome C affect the primary structure in a way not to affect the secondary and tertiary structures, which are more important for function. The amino acid that cannot be replaced without a major modification of the enzymic properties of the Cytochrome c are not altered. Thus the amino acids at locations that determine the secondary structure of protein (loops, helix or strands) are preserved while amino acids that do not contribute to the determination of secondary and tertiary structure are preferentially altered. These alterations are likely to be distributed randomly as they result from point mutations on the responsible gene and this is the single best answer of exclusion here.

Q.69. The structural proteins are involved in maintaining the shape of the cell or in the formation of matrices in the body. The shape of these proteins is: (AIPGEE 2006)

1. Globular.
2. Fibrous.
3. Stretch of beads.
4. Planar.

Ans. 2

The structural proteins are involved in maintaining the shape of a cell or in the formation of matrices in the body. The shape of these proteins is fibrous.

Collagen is the most abundant of the fibrous proteins that constitute more than 25% of the protein mass in the human body. Other prominent fibrous proteins include keratin and myosin. These proteins represent a primary source of structural strength for cells (i.e. the cytoskeleton) and tissues. Skin derives its strength and flexibility from a crisscrossed mesh of collagen and keratin fibres, while bones and teeth are buttressed by an underlying network of collagen fibres analogous to the steel strands in reinforced concrete. Collagen also is present in connective tissues such as ligaments and tendons.

Q.70. All of the following amino acids are converted to succinyl CoA except: (AIPGEE 2006)

1. **Methionine.**
2. **Isoleucine.**
3. **Valine.**
4. **Histidine.**

Ans. **4**

1. Amino acids that can be converted to **succinyl CoA**:- Methionine, isoleucine, valine and threonine are the four amino acids that can be converted to succinyl CoA.
2. Amino acids that can be converted to **alpha ketoglutarate**:- Glutamine, prolein, Arginine and Histidine are the four amino acids that can be converted to alpha ketoglutarate.
3. Amino acids that can be converted to **pyruvate**:- Alanine, serine, Glycine, cysteine, and threonine can be converted to pyruvate.
4. Amino acids that can be converted to **fumarate**:- Phenylalanine and tyrosine are the two amino acids that can be converted to fumarate.
5. Amino acid that can be converted to **acetoacetyl CoA or acetyl CoA**:- Leucine, isoleucine, lysine and tryptophan.

Q.71. The amino acid which serves as the carrier of ammonia from skeletal muscle to liver is: (AIPGEE 2006)

1. **Alanine.**
2. **Methionine.**
3. **Arginine.**
4. **Glutamine.**

Ans. **1**

The amino acid, which serves as a carrier of ammonia from skeletal muscle to liver, is alanine.

Two mechanisms are available in humans for the transport of ammonia from the peripheral tissues to the liver for its ultimate conversion to urea.

The first found in most tissues uses glutamine synthetase to combine ammonia with glutamate to form glutamine- a nontoxic transport form of ammonia. The glutamine is transported in the blood to the liver where it is cleaved by glutaminase to produce glutamate and free ammonia.

The second transport mechanism, used primarily by muscle, involves transamination of pyruvate to form alanine. Alanine is transported by the blood to the liver, where it is converted to pyruvate, again by transamination. In the liver the pathway of Gluconeogenesis can use the pyruvate to synthesize glucose, which can enter the blood and be used by muscle- a pathway called the glucose-alanine cycle.

Q.72. More than one codon coding for single amino acid: (AIIMS Nov 2006)

1. Degeneracy.

2. Frame shift mutation.

3. Transcription.

4. Mutation.

Ans. 1

If more than one codon code for a single amino acid, the genetic code is said to be degenerate. As according to the Wobble's phenomenon the last nucleotide of an anticodon does not follow Watson and crick base pairing rules.

When there is a mutation in the third nucleotide of a codon, it will not be detected by tRNA and so the amino acid sequence will not altered but only the nucleotide sequence will be altered. This is said to be silent mutation.

Q.73. All are true about proteoglycans except: (AIPGEE 2007)

1. Contains amino sugar.

2. Contains small amount of water.

3. Forms structural elements in connective tissue.

4. Condroitin sulfate is an example.

Ans. 2

Proteoglycans are proteins that contain covalently linked glycosaminoglycans eg- are hyaluronic acid, chondroitin sulfate, keratan sulfate I and II, heparin, heparan sulfate, and dermatan sulfate. A GAG is an unbranched polysaccharide made up of repeating disaccharide, one component of which is always an amino sugar (hence the name GAG).

Q.74. When urine is heated to 45^0 C a PPT is formed. When further heated to 80^0 the PPT starts redissolving. The PPT reforms on cooling. What is it? (AIPGEE 2007)

1. Albumin.

2. Globulin.

3. Bence Jones protein.

4. None.

Ans. 3

When slightly acidified urine is heated to 40^0-50^0 C and redissolve on further heating urine to boiling point. They reappear again on cooling urine to about 70^{0}C. The precipitate formed is of Bence Jones proteins. These are the light chains (k or l) of immunoglobulins that are synthesized in excess. Bence Jones proteins have a molecular weight of 20,000 or 40,000. In about 20% of the patients of multiple myeloma, Bence Jones proteins are excreted in urine, which often damages the renal tubules.

Q.75. Blackening of urine occurs in: **(AIPGEE 2007)**

1. **Alkaptonuria.**
2. **Phenyl ketonuria.**
3. **Maple syrup urine disease.**
4. **Isovaleric aciduria.**

Ans. 1

Blackening of urine occurs in the disease Alkaptonuria. This occurs when urine is exposed to sir. This occurs due to oxidation of homogentisate to benzoquinone acetate, which polymerizes and binds to connective tissue. Later, there is arthritis and connective tissue pigmentation also occurs.

Phenylketoneuria primarily causes the accumulation of phenylalanine in tissues and blood. And results in its increased excretion in urine.

During maple syrup urine disease the urine of the affected individual smells like maple syrup or burnt sugar.

During isovaleric aciduria the excretion of isovalerate is high in urine. The affected individuals exhibit a 'cheesy' odor in the breath and body fluids.

NOTES

NOTES

5

Enzymes

1. All enzymes are: Proteins.

Some RNA molecules can also act as enzymes and are called: Ribozymes.

2. The IUB classified ezymes in 6 major classes basesd on the type of reaction catalysed: Oxido reductases, transferases, hydrolases, lyases, isomerases and ligases.
3. Some enzymes contain a non-protein part called: Prosthetic group/Co-enzyme

And the protein part in enzyme called: Apoprotein/apoenzyme.

Apoenzyme + Co – enzyme: Holo enzyme.

4. Co-enzymes may be divided into two groups based on their action in the reaction:
   (a) Those which act by donating or accepting hydrogen atoms or electrons -such coenzymes are co-substrates or secondary substrates.
   (b) Those which act by transferring groups other than hydrogen i.e a particular group or radical is transferred from substrate or from coenzyme to substrate respectively. Most of them belong to vitamin B complex group.
5. The types of specificity shown by enzymes are: Absolute specificity, stereospecificity, group – specificity, optical specificity.
6. Enzymes increase the rate of chemical reaction by: Lowering the activation energy or energy barrier of the reaction.
7. The area of the enzyme where catalysis occurs is called: Active site/centre.
8. The active site of an enzyme is characterized as: A small portion of the whole enzyme to which the specific substrate is bound by non-covalent bonds for the reaction to occur or for the catalysis.
9. The hypothesis that states the active site of an enzyme is perfixed and complementary in shape to that of the substrate is called: Fischer's lock and key hypothesis
10. The hypothesis that states due to flexibility of an active site of an enzyme, it gains a complementary shape according to different substrates is called: Koshland's induced fit hypothesis

11. Enzyme found in the plasma that have a known function in the plasma are called: Functional plasma enzymes Eg. enzymes of blood coagulation.
12. Enzymes found in the plasma that have no known function in plasma are called: Non - functional plasma enzyme Eg. SGOT, SGPT whcih generally aid in diagnosis and prognosis.
13. Factors that affect tha rate of enzyme catalysed reaction are: Temperature, pH, enzyme concentration ,substrate concentration and effect of activators and inhibitors.
14. Km is defined as: Substrate concentration at half the maximum velocity and is independent of enzyme concentration.
15. Vmax is defined as: The maximum velocity obtained during the reaction.
16. The enzymes which control the whole metabolic pathway are called as: Regulatory enzymes or key enzymes or rate limiting enzymes/Allosteric enzymes.
17. An allosteric enzyme has: One catalytic site for substrate and separate allosteric site for modifier binding where the modifier binds and modulates the enzyme activity by activating or by inhibiting.
18. Increased or decreased in the number of enzyme molecules by increasing or decreasing their gene transcription is called: Induction or repression respectively.
19. Competitive inhibition: Inhibitor is structural analogue of substrate Km is increased, Vmax is unchanged.

    Non-competitive inhibition: Inhibitor has no structural resemblance to the substrate. Vmax is reduced ,Km is unchanged.

    Un-competitive inhibition: Inhibitor does not have any affinity for free enzyme.Binds to ES complex Vmax and Km both are decreased.
20. Isoenzymes are: Physically distinct forms of the same enzyme activity. They are multiple molecular forms of an enzyme.
21. Isoenzymes actually defined as: The molecular form of same enzyme which differ structurally, electrophoretically, immunologically, chemically, but carry out (catalyse) the same reaction and are products of different genes.
22. Isoenzymes have diagnostic importance.

    LDH (Lactate dehydrogenase)-5 isoenzymes. Activity increased in myocardial infarction, liver diseases.

    CK (Creatine Kinase)-3 isoenzymes.

    CK-MB is employed in: Myocardial infarction.

SOLVED QUESTIONS

Q.1. Alkaline phosphatase is produced by: (AIPGME 1994)

1. Liver

2. Bone

3. **Placenta**
4. **All of the above.**

Ans. 4

Different isoenzymes of alkaline phosphatase are seen in different tissues. Such as liver, bone, placenta etc.

Alpha-1 ALP is synthesised by epithelial cells of biliary canaliculi. Its activity is increased in obstructive jaundice and also to some extent in metastatic carcinoma of liver.

Alpha-2 heat labile ALP - is produced by hepatic cells. Its rise in activity is seen in hepatitis.

Alpha-2 heat stable ALP - is of placental origin. Found in blood in normal pregnancy.

Pre-beta ALP- is of bone origin and elevated levels are seen in bone diseases.

Gamma-ALP-originates from intestinal cells and increased activity is in ulcerative colitis.

The leucocyte alkaline phosphatase-decreased in chronic myeloid leukemia and increased in lymphomas.

Q.2.Best enzyme marker for chronic alcoholism is: (AIPGME 1999)

1. **Gamma glutamyl transferase**
2. **SGOT**
3. **SGPT**
4. **Aldolase.**

Ans. 1

Gamma glutamyl transferase (GGT) is a microsomal enzyme. Its activity is induced by alcohol, phenobarbitone and rifampicin. GGT is clinically important because of its sensitivity to detect alcohol abuse. GGT is increased in alcoholics even when other liver function tests are within normal limits. Increase in GGT level is generally proportional to the amount of alcohol intake.

Q.3. Force not acting in an enzyme substrate complex: (AIPGME 2001)

1. **Electrostatic**
2. **Covalent**
3. **Vander waals**
4. **Hydrogen.**

Ans. 3

Different theories have been proposed to explain the mechanism of enzyme action. As per Fischer's template theory substrate fits in the binding site of enzyme just as a key fits into the proper lock. Hydrogen, and ionic binding and hydrophilic interactions contribute in binding the substrate to the binding site.

Enzymes lowers decrease activation energy to enhance the rate of reaction by the processes like- substrate, strain, acid base catalysis, covalent catalysis, and entropy effects. In covalent catalysis, substrate binds to enzyme by covalent bonds. Thus the only force not acting in an enzyme substrate complex is van der waal's force.

Q.4. "All enzyme are not proteins". This statement is justified by: (AIPGME 2002)

1. **All enzyme do not follow the Michaelis Menton hypothesis**
2. **RNA act as ribozymes**
3. **Antibodies take part in the catalysis of many reactions**
4. **Metals are involved in attachment to enzyme and catalysts.**

Ans. 2

Some RNA molecules have intrinsic catalytic activity. The activity of these ribozymes often involves the cleavage of a nucleic acid . An example is the role of RNA in catalyzing the processing of the primary transcript of a gene into mature messenger RNA .

These RNA's meet all the criteria for definition of enzyme so are called as ribozymes. But RNA molecules are not proteins but still has catalytic activity (enzymatic activity). Thus all enzyme are not proteins.

Q.5. Enzymes mediating transfer of one molecule to another are: (AIPGME 2002)

1. **Transferases**
2. **Oxidases**
3. **Lyases**
4. **Peptidases.**

Ans. 1

Transferases are the enzymes that catalyse the transfer of functional groups from one molecule to another. Oxidoreductases involved in oxidations and reductions of their substrates.

Lyases-facilitate removal of small molecule from a large substrate. Peptidases - is the eg. of hydrolases which catalyze cleavage of bonds by addition of water. Peptidases degrade peptides to free amino acids.

Q.6. In which of the following conditions the level of creatinine kinase-1 increases ? (AIPGME 2004)

1. **Myocardial Ischemia**
2. **Brain Ischemia**
3. **Kidney damage**
4. **Electrical cardioversion.**

Ans. 2

There are 3 isoenzymes of creatinine kinase.

Isoenzyme. Tissue of origin

MM (CK-3) Skeletal muscle

MB (CK-2) Heart

BB(CK-1) Brain

Q.7. Enzymes that move a molecular group from one molecule to another are known as: (AIPGME 2005)

1. **Ligases**
2. **Oxido – reductases**
3. **Transferases**
4. **Dipeptidases.**

Ans. **3**

Explanation same as Q.5. Ligases-Enzymes involved in joining together two substrates.

Q.8. The enzyme not present in the skeletal muscles: **(AIIM June 1998)**

1. **Creatinine phosphokinase**
2. **Hexokinase**
3. **Phosphofructokinase**
4. **Glucose- 6-phosphatase.**

Ans. **4**

Skeletal muscles lack glucose - 6- phosphatase which is required to hydrolyse glucose -6- phosphate to free glucose. Hence glucose -6- phosphate enters into glycolytic pathway to produce lactic acid and supply ATP for muscle contraction. The energy yield from one glucose residue derived from glycogen is 3 ATP molecules, because no ATP is required for initial phosphorylation of glucose. If glycolysis starts from free glucose only 2 ATPs are produced.

Q.9. Abzyme is an: **(AIIMS 1998)**

1. **Isoenzyme**
2. **Allosteric enzyme**
3. **Abnormal enzyme**
4. **Antibody with a catalytic activity.**

Ans. **4**

Abzyme is an artificially synthesised antibody with catalytic action.

Q.10. Enzyme Ea, Eb and Ec are under allosteric control of S_2 and P_1 and P_2 respectively If Ec is defective what would occur: **(AIIMS Nov 2001)**

1. **Accumulation of S_1**
2. **Accumulation of P_1**
3. **Accumulation of S_2**
4. **Decrease of S_2.**

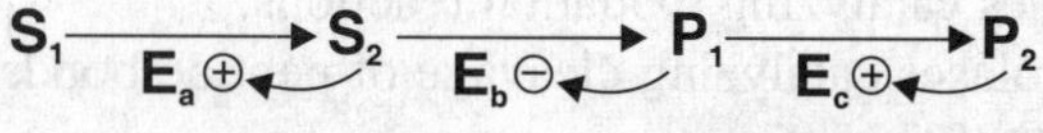

Ans. **3**

Ec is under positive control of P_2. If Ec is defective, it would block the conversion of P_1 to P_2. So p_1 gets accumulated. P_1 exerts a negative feed back effect on Eb so Eb gets inhibited. This decreases the conversion of S_2 to P_1 , so S_2 starts accumulating. Ea is under positive feedback control of S_2 and thus increases the conversion of S_1 to S_2. This leads to accumulation of S_2. The more S_2 accumulates the more enzyme Ea is activated causing increased conversion of S_1 to S_2.

Q.11. One of the following enzyme is not a protein: (AIIMS Nov 2002)

1. **DNA ase**
2. **Abzyme**
3. **EcoRI**
4. **Ribozyme.**

Ans. 4

DNAase are the enzyme capable of degrading deoxyribonucleic acid (DNA). Abzyme is an antibody with a catalytic activity and antibodies are protein in nature.

EcoRI is a restriction endonuclease that cleaves a specific double stranded DNA sequence of Ecoli. All these DNAase, Abzyme and EcoRI are enzyme or catalytic proteins but some RNA molecules having intrinsic catalytic activity are called ribozymes, that means ribozymes are RNA molecules and not the enzyme. So ribozyme is not a protein.

Q.12. Abzymes are:

1. **Carbohydrates**
2. **Ribozymes**
3. **Catalytic antibodies**
4. **Absurd enzymes.**

Ans. 3

Abzyme is artificially synthesised antibody with catalytic action

Q.13. Enzyme that catalyses the transfer of a molecular group from one molecule to another is:

1. **Oxidases**
2. **Peptidases**
3. **Transferases**
4. **Lipases.**

Ans. 3

Transferases-are the enzymes that catalyse the transfer of functional groups from one molecule to another.

Oxidases-are the enzymes catalyzing oxidation reactions.

Peptidases-are the hydrolases catalyzing cleavage of peptide bonds by addition of water.

Lipases-are the enzymes of lipid digestion.

Q.14. Multienzyme complex in humans:

1. **Fatty acid synthetase**
2. **Malonyl CoA Carboxylase**

3. Carbamoyl phosphate synthetase
4. Adenosine phospho ribosyl transferase.

Ans. 1

In humans the synthase system is a multienzyme polypeptide complex that incorporates ACP, which takes over the role of coenzyme A

Q.15. Coenzyme, in an enzymatic reaction usually functions to

1. Activate the substrate
2. Increase the active sites of apoenzyme
3. Enhance the specificity of apoenzyme
4. Accept one of the cleavage products.

Ans. 4

Coenzymes are the enzymes that contain small nonprotein molecules and metal ions that participate directly in substrate binding or catalysis or to accept one of the cleavage product.

Q.16. Aldolase is an enzyme whose substrate is:

1. Glucose-6-phosphate
2. Fructose-6-phosphate
3. Fructose
4. Fructose-1, 6-bisphosphate.

Ans. 4

During glycolysis fructose 1-6-bisphosphate is cleaved by fructose 1, 6 bisphosphate aldolase into glyceraldehyde-3-phosphate and dihydroxyacetone phosphate.

Q.17. Coenzymes are ____ organic compounds:

1. Lipoproteins
2. Proteinaceous
3. Non-Protein
4. Any of the above.

Ans. 3

Coenzymes are the enzymes that contain small nonprotein molecules and metal ions that participate directly in substrate binding or catalysis or to accept one of the cleavage product.

Q.18. Km decreases but Vmax same-enzyme is:

1. Competitive
2. Non-competitive
3. Irreversible
4. Uncompetitive

Ans. 1

A competitive inhibitor has no effects on Vmax but raises Km, the apparent Km for the substrate.

Q.19 Hormone substrate concentration affects the velocity of enzymatic action, this is known as:

1. **Zimmerman reaction**
2. **Salkowski reaction**
3. **Michales menton reaction**
4. **Lieberman-Burchard reaction.**

Ans. 3

Hormone substrate concentration affects the velocity of enzymatic action this is known as Michales menton equation.

Q.20. When the prosthetic group of an enzyme is an inorganic ion, it is called a:

1. **Cofactor**
2. **Coenzyme**
3. **Apoenzyme**
4. **Holoenzyme.**

Ans. 1

When inorganic ions present as a prosthetic group the enzyme is said to be cofactor. The most common cofactor also are metal ions. Enzymes that require a metal ion cofactor are termed metal activated enzymes to distinguish them from the metalloenzymes for which metal ions serves as prosthetic group.

Q.21. The most common enzyme deficiency in man is:

1. **Glucose-6-phosphate dehydrogenase**
2. **Glucose-6-phosphatase**
3. **Hexokinase**
4. **Glucose1, 6-diphosphatase.**

Ans. 1

Deficiency of the activity of glucose-6-phosphate dehydrogenase, is the most common of all enzymopathies. At least 100 million people are deficient in this enzyme. The disorder resulting from deficiency of glucose-6-phosphate dehydrogenase is hemolytic anemia.

Q.22. Key glycolytic enzymes:

1. **Phosphofructokinase**
2. **Hexokinase**
3. **Pyruvate kinase**
4. **Glucose 1, 6 diphosphatase.**

Ans. 1

Phosphofructokinase is the rate limiting enzyme and the major regulatory enzyme of glycolysis. AMP and fructose-2,6 bisphosphate are its activators while ATP and citrate are inhibitors.

Q.23. Which of the following is a debranching enzyme?

1. **Glycogen synthetase**
2. **Glucose-6-phosphatase**
3. **Amylo (1, 6) glycosidase**
4. **Amylo 1, 4, -1, 6 transglycosylase.**

Ans. 3

$\alpha 1 \rightarrow 6$ bonds in glycogenolysis is broken by amylo $1 \rightarrow 6$ glycosidase which is a debranching enzyme.

Q.24. Creatinine clearance, best method for estimation: (AIIMS Nov 2006)

1. **Enzyme assay.**
2. **Kinetic Jaffe.**
3. **Jaffe.**
4. **Technicon.**

Ans. 2

Actually Jaffe method is used for the estimation of creatinine clearance. During this Creatinine reacts with concentrated picric acid to form creatinine picrate which in alkaline medium, is orange yellow in color and then the intensity of the color is detected.

Jaffe method is of two types-

(a) End point assay which is used for the estimation of glucose

(b) Kinetic assay that is used for the estimation of creatinine and all type of enzymes here the change in absorbance is measured continuously. It requires automation.

Q.25. All of the following enzymes are regulated by calcium or calmodulin except: (AIPGEE 2006)

1. **Adenylate cyclase.**
2. **Glycogen synthase.**
3. **Guanyl cyclase.**
4. **Hexokinase.**

Ans. 4

Hexokinase cannot be regulated by calcium or calmodulin. It can be regulated by glucose-6- phosphate. Whereas the enzymes that are regulated by calcium or calmodulin are:-

1. Adenyl cyclase.
2. Ca^{2+} dependent protein kinases.
3. Ca^{2+}- Mg^{2+} ATPase.

4. Ca^{2+}- phospholipid dependent protein kinases.
5. Cyclic nucleotide phosphodiesterase.
6. Some cycloskeletal proteins.
7. Some ion channels (eg- Ltype calcium channels)
8. Phosphorylase kinase.
9. Phosphoprotein phosphatase 2B.
10. Some receptor (eg- NMDA type glutamate receptor)

Q.26. A common feature of all serine proteases is: (AIPGEE 2006)

1. Autocatalytic activation of zymogen precursor.

2. Tight binding of pancreatic trypsin inhibitor.

3. Cleavage of protein on the carboxyl site of serine residues.

4. Presence of serine-histidine-aspartate catalytic triad at the active site.

Ans. **4**

The common feature of all serine proteases is that they contain three amino acids –serine, histidine and aspartate which are known as catalytic triad whereas the serine proteases which functions as enzymes are chymotrypsin, elastase and trypsin. Each of these enzymes has a catalytic triad in their active sites. Serine proteases are secreted as inactive zymogens into small intestine and became active through proteolytic cleavage events, either in a subcellular compartment or in extracellular space where they are required for digestion. There are different inhibitors for different serine proteases such as –

Serine proteases	Serine protease inhibitor
Trypsin	Pancreatic trypsin inhibitor.
Chymotrypsin	Alpha-1 antichymotrypsin.
Elastase	Alpha-1 antitrypsin

Q.27. The type of enzyme inhibition (in which succinate dehydrogenase reaction is inhibited by malonate) is an example of: (AIIMS May 2006)

1. Noncompetitive.

2. Uncompetitive.

3. Competitive.

4. Allosteric.

Ans. **3**

The reaction in which malonate inhibits the succinate dehydrogenase is an example of competitive inhibition. Both succinate and its structural analogue malonate can bind to active site of succinate dehydrogenase, forming an enzyme substrate and enzyme inhibitor complex respectively.

Competitive inhibitors are similar to substrates in their structure that's why they acts by decreasing the number of free enzyme molecule available to bind substrate, i.e. to form enzyme substrate complex, and thus eventually to form product.

Q.28. All are true regarding oxygenase except: **(AIPGEE 2007)**

1. **Incorporates 1 atom of O_2 molecule.**
2. **Incorporates both the atoms of molecular O_2.**
3. **Required for reactions like hydroxylation.**
4. **Carboxylation reaction.**

Ans. **4**

Oxygenases are the group of enzymes that catalyzes the direct incorporation of oxygen into the substrate molecule. They are of two types:

1. Dioxygenases:- They are responsible for the incorporation of both the atoms of oxygen (O_2) into the substrate. Eg- homogentisate oxidase.
2. Monooxygenase:- They catalyzes the incorporation of one atom of oxygen (1/2 O_2) while the other oxygen atom is reduced to H_2O.

NOTES

NOTES

6

Vitamins and Minerals

1. Vitamins and essential minerals: Can not be synthesised by human tissues but must be included in the diet.
2. Vitamins are classified as: Water soluble and fat soluble.
3. Water soluble vitamins include: B vitamins, folic acid, niacin, pantothenic acid, biotin and vitamin C.
4. Fat soluble vitamins include: A, D, E and K.
5. Vitamins taking part in TCA cycle: Niacin, riboflavin, thiamine, pantothenic acid.
6. The vitamin required for hydroxylation of proline and lysine residues during collagen biosynthesis is: Vitamin C.
7. The vitamin serving as a donor of reducing equivalents is: Vitamin C.
8. Vitamin C is required for synthesis of: Epinephrine and norepinephrine.
9. Iron absorption from GIT is increased with the help of: Vitamin C
10. Active form of thiamine is: Thiamine pyrophosphate (TPP).
11. TPP is involved in: Decarboxylation of α - keto acids transketolase reactions.
12. Erythrocyte transketolase activity measurement is used to know: Degree of thiamine deficiency.
13. The sugar alcohol present in riboflavin is: Ribitol.
14. Biologically active forms of riboflovin are: FMN and FAD.
15. Riboflavin acts as a coenzyme for the enzymes: Oxidoreductases.
16. Deficiency of the vitamin found in newborn infants treated with phototherapy is of: Riboflavin.
17. In the body, niacin is synthesised from amino acid: Tryptophan (60 gm of tryptophan can give rise to 1 mg of niacin.).
18. Biologically active forms of niacin are: NAD^+ and $NADP^+$.
19. Plasma cholesterol is decreased by the vitamin niacin in the form of: Nicotinic acid.
20. Niacin acts as a coenzyme for the enzymes: Oxidoreductases.

21. NAD^+ and $NADP^+$ are synthesised in: Cytosol.
22. NAD^+ synthesis requires: ATP, PRPP, nicotinate and glutamine.
23. As a general rule NADH and $FADH_2$ are produecd in: Energy yielding reactions.
24. NADPH is important in: Biosynthetic reactions.
25. In maize niacin is present in form of: Niacytin (Bound form).
26. Maize niacin can be released by pretreatment with: Alkali.
27. Niacin deficiency can be caused by excessive consumption of amino acid: Leucine.
28. Consumption of sorghum causes chances of pellagra because: It has high leucine content.
29. Leucine inhibits niacin synthesis at the step of: Quinolinate phosphoribosyl transferase.
30. Active form of pyridoxine is: Pyridoxal phosphate (PLP).
31. Most of vitamin B_6 in body is present in the form of: Muscle phosphorylase.
32. PLP serves as a cofactor in: Transamination, decarboxylation and deamination reactions.
33. Antagonist drug of PLP causing pellagra like features: Isoniazid.
34. Deficiency of pyridoxine causes the deficiency of vitamin: Niacin.
35. The vitamin depleted by oral contraceptive pills is: Vitamin B_6.
36. Pantothenic acid is a precursor in the biosynthesis of: Coenzyme A.
37. Amino acid present in pantothenic acid is: Beta - alanine.
38. Biotin acts as coenzyme in: Carboxylation reactions.
39. Protein in raw egg white which destroys biotin is: Avidin.
40. Metabolites detected in urine in biotin deficiency are:
(A) Beta methyl crotonate
(B) Beta hydroxy isovalerate
(C) Beta hydroxy propionate.
41. Biotin deficiency is produced by defects in: Utilisation of the vitamin.
42. Main source of one carbon moiety in body: Serine.
43. Metabolically active form of folate, which is a coenzyme in one carbon transfer is: Tetrahydrofolate (FH_4).
44. Folate is necessary for: Proper purine nucleotide and deoxythymidylate synthesis.
45. Index of folic acid deficiency is: FIGLU (Formimino glutamic acid) excretion.
46. The commercial preparation of vitamin B_{12} is: Cyanocobalamine.
47. Two active cofactor forms of vitamin B_{12}: Methylcobalamin and 5-deoxyadenosyl cobalamine.
48. Vitamin B_{12} is transported in blood by: Transcobalamin II.
49. The intrinsic factor required for vitamin B_{12} absorption is: Glycoprotein in nature.
50. Vitamin B_{12} is stored by binding to: Transcobalamin I.
51. Sensitive index for vitamin B_{12} deficiency is: Methyl malonic aciduria, homocystinuria.
52. Deficiency of vitamin B_{12} causes impairment of synthesis of: Methionine.
53. Vitamin B_{12} function is related to: Folate metabolism.

54. The neurologic disorder in vitamin B_{12} deficiency is attributed to the: Deficiency of methionine.
55. Active form of vitamin A in body are: Retinol, retinal, retinoic acid.
56. Lipoprotein required for transport of vitamin A in plasma is: Chylomicron.
57. Vitamin A in liver is stored inside: Ito cells.
58. Retinol is processed inside the cell in: Golgi apparatus.
59. The form of vitamin A required for vision: 11 cis retinal.
60. Rhodopsin is a complex of: 11 – cis retinal + opsin.
61. Vitamin A derivative acting as a steroid hormone is: Retinol and retinoic acid.
62. Antioxidant property of vitamin A lies in: β – carotenoid.
63. Alcoholics when supplied with vitamin A are more susceptible for: Hypervitaminosis.
64. Vitamin D is derived from: 7- dehydrocholesterol.
65. Active form of vitamin D: Calcitriol (1,25- dihydroxy cholecalciferol).
66. Hydroxylation of vitamin D_3 at 25 position occurs in: Endoplasmic reticulum of hepatocytes.
67. Formation of calcitriol (1,25 dihydroxy cholecalciferol) from 25 hydroxy D_3 takes place in: Mitochondria of renal proximal convoluted tubules.
68. Most important extra renal source of calcitriol: Placenta.
69. Calcitriol is formed in: Renal tubule, bone, placenta.
70. Mode of action of calcitriol is at: Nuclear level (stimulate transcription of mRNA).
71. Fish liver oil is rich in the vitamin: Vitamin A and vitamin D.
72. Antifertility vitamin is: Vitamin E.
73. Tocopherol is transported in blood with the help of: Lipoproteins.
74. Vitamin E is stored in: Adipose tissue.
75. The mineral having sparing effect on vitamin E: Selenium.
76. The most powerful natural antioxidant is: vitamin E.
77. The greatest biological activity of vitamin E is seen in the form of: Alpha tocopherol.
78. All vitamin K are: Naphthoquinone derivatives.
79. Synthetic compound having vitamin K activity is: Menadione.
80. Coagulation factors dependent on vitamin K are: II, VII, IX, X.
81. Vitamin K is required for: Post translational modification (Formation of γ-carboxy glutamate from glutamate).
82. Vitamin K cycle occurs in: Liver.
83. The bacteria in body synthesize vitamin K in the form of: Menaquinone.
84. Commonest cause of vitamin K deficiency: Fat malabsorption.
85. Antagonistic drugs of vitamin K are: Dicoumarol and warfarin sodium.
86. All fat soluble vitamins for their absorption requires: Bile salts.

Water soluble vitamins

No . Name	Structure	Coenzyme form	Deficiency disorders
1 Ascorbic acid (c)	Related to sugar glucose	Ascorbic acid	Scurvy
2 Thiamine (B)	Substituted pyrmidine joined by a methylene bridge to a substituted thiazole	Thiamine pyrophosphate (TPP)	Beriberi, wernicke korsakoff syndrome
3 Riboflavin (B_2)	Isoalloxazine ring attached to ribitol	FAD, FMN	Ariboflavinosis
4 Niacin	Derivatives of pyridine	NAD , NADP	Pellagra
5 Pantothenic acid	Pantoic acid and β- Alanine	Coenzyme A	
6 Pyridoxine	Pyridine derivative	Pyridoxal PO_4	
7 Biotin	Imidazole derivative	Biotin	Multiple carboxylase deficiency
8 Folic acid	Pteridine + PABA + glutamic acid	Tetrahydrofolate	Megaloblastic anemia
9 Cobalamine (B_{12})	Corin ring with cobalt	5'-Deoxyadenosyl cobalamin. Methyl cobalamin	Pernicious anemia

Fat soluble vitamins

Vitamin	Structure	Function	Deficiency disorders
A	C 15 isoprenoid compound with β- ionone ring	Role in vision	Blindness
D	Steroid prohormone	Calcium metabolism	Rickets, Osteomalacia
E	Isoprenoid substituted 6 hydroxy chromanes	Free redical scavanger	
K	Polyisoprenoid substituted Naphthoquinones	Blood clotting	

ESSENTIAL MICROMINERALS (TRACE ELEMENTS)

Elements	Functions	Deficiency Disease or symptoms	Toxicity Disease of symptoms	Good sources
Chromium	Trivalent chromium, a constituent of " glucose tolerance factor ", which binds to and potentiates insulin	Impaired glucose tolerance secondary to Parenteral nutrition	--	Meat, liver, tewers, yeast, Whole grains, nuts, Cheese

Elements	Functions	Deficiency Disease or symptoms	Toxicity Disease of symptoms	Good sources
Cobalt	Required only as a constituent of vitamin B_{12}	Vitamin B_{12} deficiency	--	Food of animal origin
Copper	Constituent of oxidase enzymes: cytochrome -C, oxidase, etc, Cytosolic super oxide dismutase role in iron absorption	Anemia(hypochromic microcytic)secondary to malnutrition. Menke's syndrome	Rare,secondary to wilson's diseases	Liver
Iodine	Constituent of thyroxine triiodothyronine	Children: cretinism Adults: goiter and hypothyro-idism myxedema,	Thyrotoxicosis goiter	Iodized salt, sea food
Iron	Constituent of heme en-zymes (hemoglobin, cytochromes, ets)	Anemia (hypochromic microcytic)	Siderosis hereditary Hemochro-matosis	Red meat, liver, eggs, Iron cook ware
Manganese	Cofactor of hydrolase decarboxylase, and transferase enzymes.Gly-coprotein and proteoglycan synthesis, Mitochondrial superoxide dismutase	Unknown in humans	Inhalation poisioning produce psychotic symptoms and parkinsonism	--
Molyb-denum	Constituent of oxidase enzymes (xanthine oxidase)	Secondary to parenteral nutrition	--	--
Selenium	Constituent of glutathione peroxidase	Marginal deficiency when soil content is Low, secondary to Parentral nutrition, protein energy malnutrition	Toxic levels in some soil. Mega dose supple mentation indu-ces hair loss, dermatitis and irritability	Plants, but varies with soils content, meat
Silicon	Role in calcification of bone and in glycosaminoglycan metabolism in cartilage and connective tissue	Impairment of normal growth	Silicosis due to long term inhala-tion of silica dust	Plant food
Zinc	Cofactor of Many enzymes: lactate dehydrogenase, alkaline phosphatase, carbonic anhydratase, etc.Formation of zinc fingers in nuclear receptor for steroid–thyroid, calcitriol receptors	Hypogonadism growth failure, impaired wound healing, decreases taste and smell acuity secondary to acroderm-atitis enteropathica Parenteral nutrition	Gastrointestinal irritation, vomiting	
Fluoride	Increases hardness of bone and teeth	Dental caries, osteoporosis	Dental fluorosis	Drinking water

MINERALS: ESSENTIAL MACROMINERALS

Elements	Functions	Deficiency Diseases or symptoms	Toxicity Disease of symptoms	Source
Calcium	Constituent of bones, teeth, regulation of nerve, muscle function	Children: rickets Adults: Osteomalacia May contribute to osteoporosis	Occurs with excess absorption due to hypervitaminosis D or hypercalcemia due to hyperparathyroidism, or idiopathic hyperc-alcemis	Dairy products, beans, leafy vegetables
Phosphorus	Constituent of teeth , ATP, phosphorylated metabolic intermediates. Nucleic acids.	Children: rickets Adults:Osteomalacia	Low serum ca^{2+} Pi ratio stimulates secondary hyperparathyroidism, may lead to bone loss	Phosphate food additives
Sodium	Principal cation in extracellular fluid. Regulates plasma volume,acid base balance, Nerve and muscle function Na^+/K^+ATPase	Unknown on normal diet; secondary to injury or illness	Hypertension (insusceptible individuals)	Table Salt, salt added to prepared food
Potassium	Principal cation in intracellular fluid, nerve and muscle function Na^+/K^+ATPase	Occurs secondary to illness, injury, or diuretic therapy, muscular weakness, paralysis, mental confusion	Cardiac arrest small bowel ulcers	Vegetables fruit buts
Chloride	Fluid and electrolyte balance: gastric fluid; chloride shifts in HCO^-_3 transport in erythrocytes	Infants fed salt-free formula, Secondary to vomiting, diuretic therapy, renal disease	--	Table salt
Magnesium	Constituent of bones, teeth enzyme co-fact or (kinases ,etc)	Secondary to malabsorption or diarrhea, alcoholism	Depressed deep tendon reflexes and respiration	Leafy green vegetable (containing chlorophyl)

SOLVED QUESTIONS

Q.1. The vitamin used for post translational modification of glutamic acid to γ carboxy glutamate is: (AIPGME 1994)

1. **Vitamin D**
2. **Vitamin E**

3. **Vitamin A**
4. **Vitamin K.**

Ans. 4

Vitamin K is necessary for coagulation. Factors dependent on vitamin k are factors II (prothrombin), VII (SPCA), IX (Christmas factor) and X (Stuart – prower factor). All these factors are synthesised by the liver as inactive zymogens. They undergo post translational modification; gamma carboxylation of glutamic acid residues. The gamma carboxy glutamic acid synthesis requires vitamin k as a cofactor. Vitamin D is related with calcium metabolism, vitamin E is the most powerful natural antioxidant, vitamin A is associated with visual cycle

Q.2. Thiamine is essential for: **(AIPGME 1995)**

1. **Isocitrate dehydrogenase**
2. **Succinate dehydrogenase**
3. **Pyruvate dehydrogenase**
4. **Acetyl CoA synthetase.**

Ans. 3

Thiamine is used as a coenzyme for oxidative decarboxylation of α-keto acids (eg pyruvate and α-ketoglutarate)

$$\text{Pyruvate} \xrightarrow[\text{TPP}]{\text{Pyruvate dehydrogenase complex}} \text{Acetyl CoA}$$

$$\alpha\text{-ketoglutarate} \xrightarrow[\text{TPP}]{\alpha\text{-ketoglutarate dehydrogenase complex}} \text{Succinyl co A}$$

Isocitrate dehydrogenase requires niacin coenzyme ie. NAD^+ succinate dehydrogenase needs riboflavin coenzyme i.e FAD.

Q.3. Which vitamin is necessary for coenzyme A synthesis: **(AIPG 1995)**

1. **Pantothenic acid**
2. **Ascorbic acid**
3. **Biotin**
4. **Pyridoxin.**

Ans. 1

Synthesis of coenzyme A

Pantothenic acid +ATP ⟶ 4-Phospho pantothenic acid + ADP

4-Phospho pantothenic acid + cysteine ⟶ 4-Phospho pantothenyl cysteine

4- Phosphopantothenyl cysteine ⟶ 4 - Phosphopantotheine + CO_2

4- Phosphopantotheine + ATP ⟶ Dephospho CoA + PPi

Dephospho CoA + ATP ⟶ Coenzyme A + ADP

Structure of coenzyme A

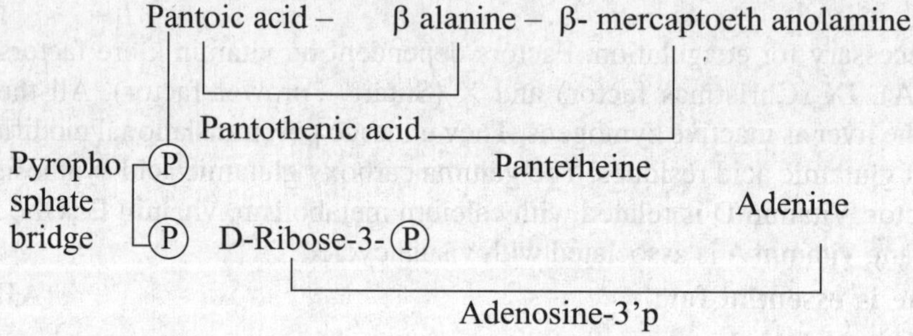

Coenzyme A is a nucleotide

Q.4. Cobalt forms a component of which vitamin:

1. **Biotin**
2. **Vitamin B_{12}**
3. **Vitamin A**
4. **Tocopherol.**

Ans. **2**

Central portion of vitamin B_{12} consists of four reduced and extensively substituted " pyrrole rings " surrounding a single cobalt atom (Co). This central structure is called: " corrin ring" system. When cyanide is bound to cobalt atom is called as cyanocobalamine.

Cobalt is required only as a constituent of vitamin B_{12} . While biotin, vitamin A and tocopherol has no metal as constituent part

Q.5. Biotins act on: **(AIPGME 1996)**

1. Carboxylation
2. Oxidative phosphorylation
3. Oxidative deamination.
4. Transmethylation.

Ans. **1**

Biotin acts as co-enzyme for carboxylation reactions. Biotin is the prosthetic group of certain enzymes (carboxylases) that catalyse CO_2 transfer reaction. In the first step, biotin first accepts CO_2 and gets converted to carboxybiotin which then transfers CO_2 to the substrate.

Q.6. Vitamin B_{12} is absorbed in the: **(AIPG 1996)**

1. **Stomach**
2. **Duodenum**
3. **Ileum**
4. **Colon.**

Ans. 3

Vitamin B_{12} is absorbed from Ileum; for its proper absorption it requires presence of HCL and intrinsic factor of castle (IF). Intrinsic factor binds B_{12} for transport through the intestinal lumen to the absorptive site in the ileum. IF-B_{12} complex is attached with specific receptors on mucosal cells. The whole complex is internalised. The IF is digested inside the mucosal cell and B_{12} is transported to the circulation.

Q.7. Vitamin required for post translational modification of coagulants is: (AIPGME 1997)

1. **Vitamin A**
2. **Vitamin C**
3. **Vitamin B_6**
4. **Vitamin K.**

Ans. 4

Vitamin K is necessary for coagulation. Factors dependent on vitamin K are factors II (Prothrombin), VII (SPCA), IX (christmas factor) and X (Stuart-prower factor.) All these factors are synthesised by the liver as inactive zymogens. They undergo post-translational modificaton. gamma carboxylation of glutamic acid residues. The gamma carboxy glutamic acid synthesis requires vitamin K as a cofactor.

Vitamin A is required for visual cycle.

Vitamin C is involved in reversible oxidation reduction reactions. hydroxylation of proline and lysine during collagen formation. It has antioxidant property also.

Vitamin B_6 acts as a coenzyme for transamination, decarboxylation reactions. Also involved in heme synthesis and niacin production.

Q.8. Thiamine acts as a cofactor in: (AIPGME 1999)

1. **Conversion of pyruvate to acetyl COA**
2. **Transamination reactions**
3. **Oxidation in respiratory chain**
4. **Conversion of pyridoxal to pyridoxal phosphate**

Ans. 1

Thiamine acts as a cofactor in oxidative decarboxylation of alpha keto acids (eg.pyruvate and alpha ketoglutarate)

$$\text{Pyruvate} \xrightarrow[\text{TPP}]{\text{Pyruvate dehydrogenase complex}} \text{Acetyl COA}$$

$$\alpha\text{-Ketoglutarate} \xrightarrow[\text{TPP}]{\alpha\text{-Ketoglutarate dehydrogenase complex}} \text{Succinyl CoA}$$

For transamination reactions, vitamin B_6 (Pyridoxal phosphate) acts as a coenzyme.

For oxidation in respiratory chain NAD^+ (niacin) and FAD (riboflavin) coenzymes are required for phosphorylation of pyridoxal to pyridoxal phosphate ATP is required.

Q.9. The similarity between vitamin C and vitamin K is: **(AIPGME 2000)**

1. **Both help in conversion of proline to hydroxyproline**
2. **Both help in post translational modification**
3. **Both have anti infective activity**
4. **Both are involved in coagulation cascade.**

Ans. **2**

Vitamin C is required for post translational modification of proline and lysine to hydrxyproline and hydrxylysine in collagen synthesis.

Vitamin K is needed for post translational modification: gamma carboxylation of glutamate residues during synthesis of active clotting factors.

Thus both help in post translational modification.

Its only vitamin C but not vitamin K that helps in conversion of proline to hydroxyproline.

Both vitamins are not involved in coagulation cascade only vitamin K is required.

Q.10. Thiamine level is best monitored by: **(AIPGME 2002)**

1. **Transketolase level in blood**
2. **Thiamine level in blood**
3. **G6PD activity**
4. **Reticulocytosis.**

Ans. **1**

As thiamine acts as a cofactor for transketolase, its deficiency is diagnosed by measuring transketolase level in blood (in erythrocytes). An increase in erythrocyte transketolase activity is observed upon addition of thiamine pyrophosphate in thiamine deficient persons.

Q.11. Vitamin B_{12} and folic acid supplementation in megaloblastic anemia leads to the improvement of anemia due to: **(AIPGME 2002)**

1. **Increased DNA synthesis in bone marrow**
2. **Increased hemoglobin production**
3. **Erythroid hyperplasia**
4. **Increased iron absorption.**

Ans. **1**

Vitamin B_{12} and folic acid metabolism are related with each other. Vitamin B_{12} is a coenzyme in the conversion of methyltetrahydrofolate to tetrahydrofolate (active form of folic acid). So Vitamin B_{12} deficiency produces folic acid deficiency i.e tetrahydrofolate is not synthesized. Tetrahydrofolate is necessary for purine and pyrimidine synthesis which are required for nucleic acid (DNA, RNA) synthesis. Deficiency of Vitamin B_{12} and folic acid thus impairs DNA synthesis preventing cell division as well as formation of the nucleus of new RBCs. This causes megaloblastic anemia.

So supplementation of vitamin B_{12} and folic acid corrects both the deficiencies there by causing increased DNA synthesis in bone marrow and improvement of anemia.

Q.12. A middle aged woman on oral contraceptives for many years, developed neurological symptoms such as depression, irritability, nervousness and mental confusion. Her hemoglobin level was 8 g/dl. Biochemical investigations revealed that she was excreting highly elevated concentrations of xanthurenic acid in urine. she also showed high levels of triglycerides and cholesterol in serum. All of the above findings are most probably related to Vitamin B_6 deficiency caused by prolonged oral contraceptive use except: (AIPGME 2004)

1. **Increased urinary xanthurenic acid excretion**
2. **Neurological symptoms by decreased synthesis of biogenic amines**
3. **Decreased hemoglobin level**
4. **Increased triglyceride and cholesterol level.**

Ans. 4

In women taking oral contraceptives and steroids, vitamin B_6 deficiency is seen. In Vitamin B_6 deficiency, PLP dependent enzymes function poorly. So serotonin, epinephrine, noradrenalin and gamma amino butyric acid (GABA) are not produced properly resulting in neurological symptoms. Vitamin B_6 (PLP) acts as a coenzyme for ALA synthase, the rate limiting enzyme of heme synthetic pathway. In vitamin B_6 deficiency, there is reduced activity of this enzyme resulting in hypochromic microcytic anemia. The enzyme kynureninase required for niacin synthesis is a PLP dependent enzyme. It catalyses conversion of 3- hydroxy kynurenine to 3- hydroxy anthranilic acid. In Vitamin B_6 deficiency kynurenine can not be metabolised further and gets diverted to conversion into xanthurenic acid which is excreted through urine. PLP is involved in the formation of ceramide and sphingolipids so PLP deficiency hampers their metabolism.

Q.13. Both vitamin K and C are involved in: (AIPGME 2005)

1. **The synthesis of clotting factors**
2. **Post translational modifications**
3. **Antioxidant mechanisms**
4. **The microsomal hydroxylation reactions.**

Ans. 2

Explanation same as Q.9

Q.14. Vitamin K is needed for which of these post translational modification processes: (AIIMS May 2001)

1. **Methylation**
2. **Carboxylation**
3. **Hydroxylation**
4. **Transketolation.**

Ans. 2

Vitamin K is needed for gamma carboxylation of glutamic acid residues in the synthesis of active clotting factors. Vitamin K functions as a coenzyme for carboxylase.

Q.15. Thiamine is not used in which of the following reactions: (AIIMS May 2001)

1. **Lactate to pyruvate**
2. **Alpha ketoglutarate to succinyl CoA**
3. **Glucose to pentose**
4. **Oxidative decarboxylation of alpha keto amino acids.**

Ans. 1

Conversion of lactate to pyruvate and pyruvate to lactate is a reversible oxidation - reduction reaction. It is catalysed by the enzyme lactate dehydrogenase. Reducing equivalents are accepted or donated by niacin coenzyme ie NAD^+.

Thiamine is used as a coenzyme in two types of reaction–

(1) Transketolase reaction (HMP shunt) which involves interconversions of sugars. It is a pathway for production of pentose from glucose.

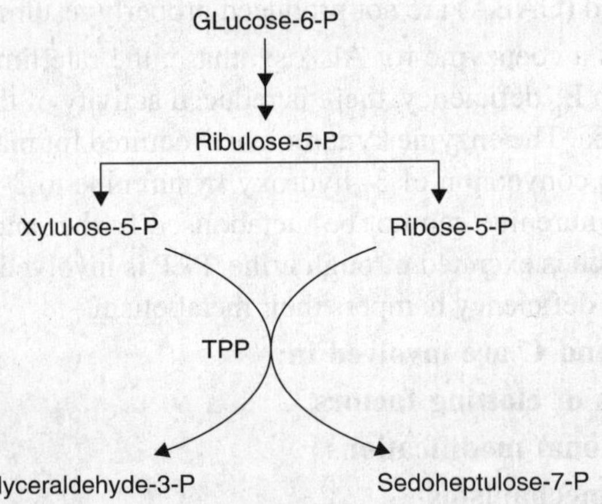

(2) Oxidative decarboxylation of alpha keto acid

$$\text{Pyruvate} \xrightarrow[\text{TPP}]{\text{Pyruvate dehydrogenase Complex}} \text{Acetyl CoA}$$

$$\text{Alpha ketoglutarate} \xrightarrow[\text{TPP}]{\alpha\text{-KGA dehydrogenase complex}} \text{Succinyl CoA}$$

Q.16. The activity of the following enzyme is affected by biotin deficiency: (AIIMS 2003)

1. **Transketolse**
2. **Dehydrogenase**
3. **Oxidase**
4. **Carboxylase.**

Ans. 4

Explanation same as Q.5

Q.17. Which of the following combinations of biologically active molecules does vitamin A consists of ? (AIIMS May 2004)

1. **Retinol, retinal and retinoic acid**
2. **Retinol, retinal and tetrahydro folate**
3. **Retinal, conjugase and retinoic acid**
4. **PABA, retinal and retinaldehyde.**

Ans. 1

All the compounds with vitamin A activity are referred to as retinoids. The different compounds with vitamin A activity are retinol (vitamin A alcohol), retinal (vitamin A aldehyde) and retinoic acid (vitamin A acid), with corresponding functional groups on the polyisoprenoid side chain.

Q.18. Thiamine deficiency can be diagnosed by measuring;

1. **Thiamine levels in blood**
2. **Alkaline phosphatase levels in blood**
3. **Transketolase activity in RBC**
4. **Plasma pyruvate and lactate levels.**

Ans. 3

Explanation same as Q.10

Q.19. Pantothenic acid is an integral component of:

1. **NAD**
2. **Cobalamine**
3. **Folic acid**
4. **Coenzyme A**

Ans. 4

Structure of coenzyme A is

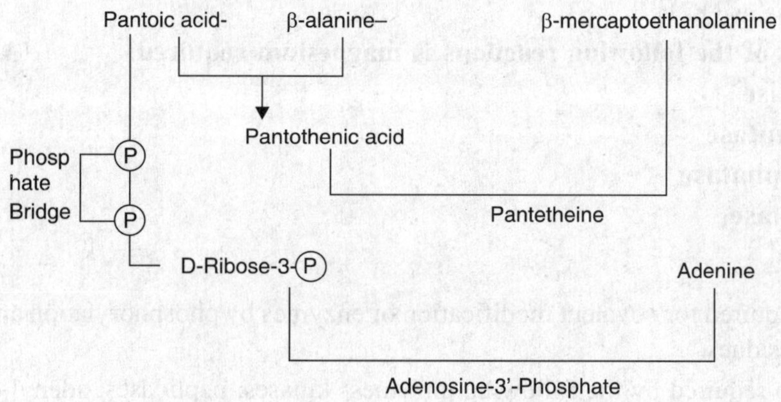

Q.20. Thiamine deficiency would lead to defects in:

1. **Conversion of pyruvate to acetyl CoA**
2. **Electron transphatase**
3. **Hydrogen accepting coenzymes**
4. **Collagen**

Ans. **1**

The coenzyme form of thiamine is thiamine pyrophosphate. It is used in oxidative decarboxylation of alpha keto acids eg. Pyruvate decarboxylase, a component of the pyruvate dehydrogenase complex which catalyses conversion of pyruvate to acetyl CoA So thiamine deficiency leads to defect in the conversion of pyruvate to acetyl CoA

Q.21. Cofactor associated with the enzyme glutathione peroxidase is: **(AIPG 96)**

1. **Zinc**
2. **Cadmium**
3. **Molybdenum**
4. **Selenium.**

Ans. **4**

In mammals, glutathione peroxidase is the important selenium containing enzyme . Mammalian glutathione peroxidase contains 4 polypeptide chains, each having one selenocysteine residue. RBC contains good quantity of glutathione peroxidase.

Q.22. Selenium is cofactor for: **(AIPGME 1998)**

1. **Glutathione peroxidase**
2. **Glutathione reductase**
3. **Glutathione synthetase**
4. **Glutathione dehydrogenase.**

Ans. **1**

Explanation same as Q.21

Q.23. In which of the following reactions is magnesium required: **(AIPGME 2002)**

1. **ATPase**
2. **Dismutase**
3. **Phosphatase**
4. **Aldolase.**

Ans. **3**

Magnesium is required for covalent modification of enzymes by phosphorylation and dephosphorylation of seryl residues.

Mg^{++} is also required by the following enzymes kinases, peptidases, adenyl cyclase, ribonuclease, carboxylase transketolase.

Q.24. Which of the following elements is known to influence the body's ability to handle oxidative stress? (AIPG 2004)

1. **Calcium**
2. **Iron**
3. **Postassium**
4. **Selenium.**

Ans. 4

Selenium acts as a non-specific intracellular antioxidant. This action of Se is complementary to vitamin E. Availability of vitamin E reduces the Se requirement selenium protects animals from carcinogenic chemicals. Selenium also binds Cd, Hg and other heavy metals and mitigates their toxic effects. Glutathione peroxidase a selenium containing enzyme is also involved in antioxidant function.

Q.25. Biological role of metallothioneins is to sequester harmful metal ions. These bind: (AIIMS May 2004)

1. Cd^{++}, Cu^{++} **and** Zn^{++}
2. Al^{+++}, Hg^{++} **and** NH_4^+
3. Pt^{++}, As^{+++}, **and** PO_4^-
4. Fe^{+++}, Na^+ **and** k^+

Ans. 1

Metallothioneins are a group of small proteins found in the cytosol of cells, Particularly of liver, kidney and intestine. They have a high content of cysteine and can bind copper, zinc, cadmium and mercury. The – SH groups of cysteine are involved in binding the metals.

Q.26. Pantothenic acid acts on:

1. **NADP**
2. **NADPH**
3. **FAD**
4. **CoA.**

Ans. 4

Pantothenic acid has a central role in acyl group metabolism when acting as the pantetheine functional moiety of coenzyme A or acyl carrier protein (ACP)

Q.27. Magnesium is needed for the activity of which enzyme:

1. **Phosphatase**
2. **Aldolase**
3. **Dismutase**
4. **ATPase.**

Ans. 1

Explanation same as Q.23

Q.28. Deficiency of thiamine causes:

1. **Beri Beri**
2. **Scurvy**
3. **Night blindness**
4. **Rickets.**

Ans. **1**

Thiamine deficiency causes peripheral nerve damage (beri beri) or central nervous system lesions (Wernicke- Korsakoff syndrome)

Q.29. The metabolism of 'FIGLU' is dependent on:

1. **Niacin**
2. **Thiamine**
3. **Biotin**
4. **Folic acid.**

Ans. **4**

During Histidine metabolism formimino group transfer to THF forms glutamate, then α-ketoglutarate. In folic acid deficiency, group transfer is impaired and FIGLU is excreted.

Excretion of FLGLU following a dose of histidine thus has been used to detect folic acid deficiency.

Q.30. Which is a pro vitamin or vitamin that has antioxidant properties?

1. **Beta carotene**
2. **Vitamin E**
3. **Vitamin C**
4. **Vitamin D**

Ans. **2**

The main function of vitamin E is a chain-breaking, free trapping antioxidant in cell membranes and plasma lipoproteins.

Q.31. Deficiency of which vitamin is not known in newborn?

1. **C**
2. **D**
3. **E**
4. **K.**

Ans. **3**

vitamin E defiency is unknown in humans. Some premature infants are born with inadequate reserves of the vitamin.

Q.32. Biotin is essential for:

1. **Translation**
2. **Carboxylation**
3. **Hydroxylation**
4. **Transamination**

Ans. 2

Biotin functions to transfer CO_2 in a number of carboxylation reactions.

Q.33. Which of the following vitamin act as a respiratory catalyst?

1. **B_2**
2. **Pyridoxine**
3. **B_{12}**
4. **C**

Ans. 1

Flavin coenzymes carry electrons in oxidation reduction reactions. They include the mitochondrial respiratory chain, key enzymes in fatty acids and amino acid oxidation, and the citric acid cycle. Because of this, flavin oxidases make a significant contribution to the total oxidant stress of the body.

Q.34. The reaction inhibited in thiamine deficiency is:

1. **Pyruvate to acetyl CoA**
2. **Citrate to alpha ketoglutarate**
3. **Succinyl CoA to fumarate**
4. **None**

Ans. 1

The central role of thiamine diphosphate in pyruvate dehydrogenase means that in deficiency of thiamine there is a impaired conversion of pyruvate to acetyl COA.

Q.35. A vitamin which functions as reducing agent is?

1. **B_{12}**
2. **Vitamin C**
3. **Nicotinamide**
4. **Folate.**

Ans. 2

Vitamin C has specific roles in the Cu containing hydroxylases and the α- ketoglutarate linked iron containing hydroxylases. It also increases the activity of a number of other enzymes in vitro, though this has a non-specific reducing action.

Q.36. Vitamin used for post translational modification of glutamic acid to gamma carboxy glutamate is

1. **A**

2. D
3. B
4. K

Ans. 4

Viamin K is the factor for the carboxylation of glutamate residues in the post synthetic modification of proteins to form the unusual amino acids γ- carboxy glutamate which chelates the calcium ion.

Q.37. Which of the following is the component of the visual pigment rhodopsin? (AIIMS Nov 2005)

1. **β-carotene.**
2. **Retinal.**
3. **Retinol.**
4. **Retinoic acid.**

Ans. 2

Retinal is derived from the oxidation of retinol. Both of them can readily be interconvertible. Retinal is the only component of visual pigment rhodopsin whereas, the retinoic acid derived from oxidation of dietary retinol, mediates most of the actions of the retinoids such as maintenance of reproduction, promotion of growth, gene expression except for vision which depends on retinal, the aldehyde derivative of retinol.

Q.38. Vitamin is stored mainly as retinol esters in: (AIIMS Nov 2005)

1. **Kidney.**
2. **Muscle.**
3. **Liver.**
4. **Retina.**

Ans. 3

Vitamin is stored as retinol esters in liver. Retinol esters present in the diet are hydrolyzed in the intestinal mucosa, releasing retinol and free fatty acids and secreted as chylomicrons in to the lymphatic system. These chylomicrons are taken up by, and stored in the liver.

Q.39. Vitamin B_{12} acts as coenzyme to which one of the following enzymes: (AIPGEE 2006)

1. **Isocitrate dehydrogenase.**
2. **Homocysteine methyltransferase.**
3. **Glycogen synthase.**
4. **Glucose- 6- phosphate dehydrogenase.**

Ans. 2

Vitamin B_{12} is required as a coenzyme to homocysteine methyl transferase involved in the synthesis of methionine from homocysteine.

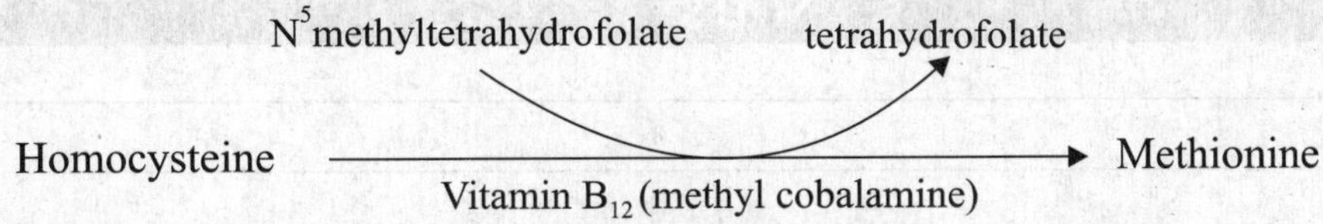

Q.40. Transport of ascorbic acid to lens is done by? **(AIPGEE 2007)**

1. **Myoionositol.**
2. **Choline.**
3. **Taurine.**
4. **Na-K ATPase.**

Ans. **1**

Q.41. Biotin is useful in: **(AIPGEE 2007)**

1. **Alpha keto acid carboxylase deficiency.**
2. **Multiple carboxylase deficiency.**
3. **Decarboxylation reactions.**
4. **All of the above.**

Ans. **2**

Biotin is useful in multiple carboxylase deficiency. As it is involved in various carboxylation reactions. It functions to transfer CO_2 in a small number of Carboxylation reactions. A holocarboxylase synthetase acts on a lysine residue of the apoenzymes of acetyl CoA carboxylase, pyruvate carboxylase, propionyl CoA carboxylase, or methyl crotonyl CoA carboxylase to react with free biotin to form the biocytin residue of the holoenzyme. The reactive intermediate is 1-N carboxybiotin, formed from bicarbonate in an ATP dependent reaction. The carboxyl group is then transferred to the substrate for Carboxylation.

NOTES

7 Hormones

1. The secretions of the endocrine glands (ductless glands) are: Hormones.
2. Hormones are defined as the organic/chemical substances produced in one part of body, enter the circulation and carried to distant target organs and tissues to control their metabolic and biological activities.
3. Classification of hormones: Two types of classification.

   Type 1 classification based on chemical nature–

   (a) Steroid hormones – Steroid in nature. Eg. glucocorticoids, mineralocorticoids and sex hormones.

   (b) Amino acid derivatives– Derived from amino acid tyrosine. Eg. Epinephrine, norepinephrine and thyroid hormones.

   (c) Protein/Peptide hormones – Eg. Insulin, glucagons, etc.

   Type 2 classification

Group 1 Hormones: That binds to intracellular receptor. Eg. Steroid hormones, thyroid hormones.

   Group 2 Hormones: That bind to cell surface receptors. Mediate their action through second messengers.

   (a) Second messenger is cAMP – Eg. Catecholamines, ACTH, ADH, calcitonin,CRH, FSH, LH, MSH, TSH, PTH, hcG

   (b) Second messenger is cGMP – Eg. Atrial natriuretic factor (ANF), nitric oxide (NO).

   (c) Second messenger is calcium or phosphatidylinositol or both. Eg.TRH, GnRH, oxytocin, ADH, angiotensin II

   (d) Second messenger is kinase or phosphatase cascade. Eg. Insulin, prolactin.
4. The hormone – receptor complex activates the regulatory component of the protein: G-protein or nucleotide regulatory protein.
5. The G-protein is a: Peripheral membrane protein consisting of alpha, beta and gamma subunits.

	Group 1 Hormones	Group 2 Hormones
Solubility	Lipophilic	Hydrophilic
Transport Proteins	Yes	No
Plasma half life	Long (hours to day)	Short (minutes)
Receptors	Intracellular	Plasma membrane
Mediators	Receptor – Hormone Complex	cAMP, cGMP

6. Adenylate cyclase is stimulated by: GTP dependent protein – Gs.
7. Adenylate cyclase is inhibited by: GTP dependent protein – Gi.
8. In mammalian cells, cAMP binds to an enzyme: Protein kinase.
9. Hormones increasing the level of cAMP by stimulation of adenylate cyclase in adipose tissue: ACTH, TSH, glucagon, epinephrine, MSH, vasopressin.
10. cAMP serves as a messenger for the action of: Polypeptide hormones.
11. Hormone receptors with no known ligand are called: Orphan receptors.
12. In relation to carbohydrate metabolism; Growth hormone antagonizes the action of: Insulin.
13. More than one physiologically potent polypeptides are present in the hormone: Proopiomelanocortin.
14. Proopiomelanocortin (POMC) is from: Anterior and intermediate lobe of pituitary.
15. Beta endorphin is secreted from: Intermediate lobe of pituitary.
16. The number of amino acids in ADH and oxytocin are: 9 amino acids.
17. Most important target cell for ADH: Collecting duct and DCT.
18. Normal $T_4 : T_3$ ratio in thyroglobulin is: 7 : 1.
19. $T_4 : T_3$ ratio decreases in: Iodine deficiency.
20. Storage form of thyroid hormones: Thyroglobulin.
21. The binding proteins for thyroid hormones: Thyroxin binding globulin (TBG) and thyroxin binding prealbumin (TBPA).
22. The Oxidation of iodide is inhibited by: Thiourea drugs.
23. Drugs competing with T_3 and T_4 for binding to TBG: Phenytoin and salicylate.
24. Tissues involved in peripheral metabolism of parathyroid: Kidney, liver.
25. The principal site of proteolysis of parathyroid hormone: Kupffer cells of liver.
26. The only hormone that increases calcium absorption across intestinal mucous: Calcitriol.
27. PTH level is directly proportional to: Serum calcium level.
28. Predominant glucocorticoid in humans: Cortisol.
29. The biologically active fraction of cortisol is: Unbound or free fraction.
30. Most common enzyme deficient in congential adrenal hyperplasia: 21- Hydroxylase.
31. Monoamine oxidase enzyme is found in highest concentration in: Liver.
32. The major androgen precursor produced by adrenal cortex: Dehydroepiandrosterone (DHEA).
33. Testosterone is produced from: Leydig cells.

34. The primary estrogen of ovarian origin is: 17 Beta oestradiol.
35. Major source of estrogens in post menopausal women: Aromatization of adrenal androgens.
36. Major progesterone metabolite found in urine: Pregnandiol –20–glucuronide.
37. Major source of progesterone in early pregnancy: Corpus luteum.
38. Glucagon increases the level of cAMP in: Liver but not in muscle.
39. The first protein to be sequenced was: Insulin.
40. High concentration of zinc is found in the pancreatic: β – cell.
41. Polypeptide sequence of insulin was first given by: Sanger.
42. Nitric oxide acts as a neurotransmitter in: Peripheral nerves.
43. Erythropoetin is produced in: Kidney.
44. A polypeptide of 22 amino–acid from G.I.T. that functions to control the G.I. muscle is: Motilin.

SOLVED QUESTIONS

Q.1. Cylic GMP act on: **(AIPGME 1997)**

1. **Insulin**
2. **Thyroxin**
3. **Atrial natriuretic peptide**
4. **Growth hormone.**

Ans. **3**

Second messenger for atrial natriuretic peptide is c-GMP. Thyroxine bind to intracellular receptor. For insulin second messenger is kinase or phosphatase cascade

Q.2. The hormone using an enzyme receptor for its action: **(AIPGME 2000)**

1. **Insulin**
2. **Steroid**
3. **Oestrogen**
4. **Thyroxine.**

Ans. **1**

Steroid hormones, oestrogen and thyroid hormones bind to intracellular receptor. Insulin has tyrosine kinase as a receptor for its action .

Q.3. All are actions of insulin except: **(AIPGME 2000)**

1. **Gluconeogenesis**
2. **Glycolysis**
3. **Glycogenesis**
4. **Lipogenesis.**

Ans. **1**

Insulin lowers the blood glucose level. Thus it favors glycolysis, glycogen synthesis (Glycogenesis) and lipid synthesis. While it inhibits gluconeogenesis.

Q.4. Insulin does not facilitate glucose uptake in the following except:

1. Liver

2. Heart

3. RBC

4. Kidney.

Ans. **2**

Insulin facilitate glucose uptake with the help of glucose transporter 4 (GLUT 4) . It mediates glucose uptake only in –

(a) Muscle – skeletal muscle and cardiac muscle (Heart)

(b) Adipose tissue.

Q.5. Which of the following is a membrane bound enzyme that catlayzes the formation of cAMP from ATP: (AIPGME 2004)

1. Tyrosine kinase

2. Polymerase

3. ATP synthase

4. Adenylate cyclase.

Ans. **4**

The extracellular messenger, the hormone (H) combines with the specific receptor on the plasma membrane. This complex stimulates the G protein, which carries the excitation signal to adenylate cyclase which converts ATP to cAMP

Q.6. Which of the following substances acts to increase the release of Ca^{++} from endoplasmic reticulum: (AIPGME 2004)

1. Inositol triphosphate

2. Parathyroid hormone

3. 1,25- dihydroxy cholecalciferol

4. Diacylglycerol.

Ans. **1**

Phospholipase C hydrolyzes the phosphatidyl inositol bishosphate to diacylglycerol and inositol triphosphate can release Ca^{++} from intracellular stores such as from endolasmic reticulum and from sarcoplasmic reticulum.

Q.7. A small Ca^{++} binding protein that modifies the activity of many enzymes and other proteins in response to changes of Ca^{++} concentration is known as:

1. Cycline

2. Calmodulin

3. **Collagen**
4. **Kinesin.**

Ans. 2

Calmodulin, the calcium dependent regulatory protein within the cell has four calcium binding sites. when calcium binds there is a conformational change to the calmodulin, which has a role in regulating various kinases.

Q.8. The following hormone does not have any intracellular receptor:

(AIPGME nov 2002)

1. **Vitamin D3**
2. **Cortisone**
3. **Adrenaline**
4. **Thyroxine.**

Ans. 3

Hormones that bind to intracellular receptors are glucocorticoids, mineralocorticoids , estrogens, progesterone ,androgens, calcitriol and thyroxine. Adrenaline bind with cell surface receptors with c AMP as the second messenger.

Q.9. Insulin increases the activities of all of the following enzymes except:

(AIPGME 2004)

1. **Glucokinase**
2. **Pyruvate carboxylase**
3. **Glycogen synthase**
4. **Acetyl co A carboxylase.**

Ans. 2

Insulin lowers blood glucose level that means it facilitates glucose utilization. Thus it increases the activities of following enzyme. Glucokinase –Glycolysis (energy production). Glycogen synthase - Glycogenesis (storage form). Acetyl co A carboxylase – lipogenesis (storage as lipids). Insulin inhibits gluconeogenesis by inhibiting pyruvate carboxylase.

Q.10. Not produced in Adrenaline synthesis pathway:

1. **DOPA**
2. **Dopamine**
3. **Nor adrenaline**
4. **Tyramine.**

Ans. 4

The adrenalin synthesis involves the conversion of L-Tyrosine to Dopa which on decarboxylation gets converted to dopamine and then to noradrenalin and adrenalin respectively.

Q.11. Insulin promotes transport of glucose in which of these:

1. **Hepatocytes**
2. **Muscles**
3. **RBC**
4. **Adipose tissue.**

Ans. **1**

In addition to the direct effects of hyperglycemia in enhancing the uptake of glucose into the liver, the hormone insulin plays a central role in regulating blood glucose.

Q.12. Norepinephrine is converted to epinephrine by:

1. **O-methylation**
2. **N-methylation**
3. **Dopamine hydroxylase**
4. **Dopa decarboxylase.**

Ans. **2**

In the adrenal medulla, phenylethanolamine N-methyltransferase utilizes S-adenosylmethionine to methylate the primary amine of norepinephrine, forming epinephrine.

Q.13. Calcium as a second messenger in hormone action involves all except:

1. **cGMP**
2. **Na^+/Ca^+ exchange pump**
3. **Protein kinase**
4. **Phosphatidyl inositol.**

Ans. **1**

Ca is as intracellular messanger of hormone action with phosphatidyl ionositols. It activates sevaral hormones. As the prolonged elevation of Ca^{2+} in the cell is very toxic. A Na^+ / Ca^{2+} exchange mechanism that has high capacity but low affinity pumps Ca^{2+} out of the cells.

Q.14. All are second messengers, except:

1. **c-AMP**
2. **Calcium**
3. **m-RNA**
4. **Phosphatidyl inositol.**

Ans. **3**

The hormones that bind to the cell surface receptors are called second messengers. This group includes cAMP, cGMP, Ca^{2+} , phosphatidyl ionositol, kinase and phosphatase.

Q.15. Precursor of testosterone is:

1. **Estrone**
2. **Cholesterol**

3. **Cortisol**
4. **Aldosterone**

Ans. 2

The immediate precursor of the gonadal steroids, as for the adrenal steroids, is cholesterol.

Q.16. Rate limiting step in adrenaline synthesis is conversion of:

1. **Tyrosine to dopa**
2. **Phenylalanine to tyrosine**
3. **Dopa to dopamine**
4. **Dopamine to norepinephrine**

Ans. 1

Tyrosine is the immediate precursor of catecholamines, and tyrosine hydroxylase is the rate limiting enzyme in catecholamines biosynthesis. Tyrosine hydroxylase is found in both soluble and particle bound forms only in tissues that synthesize catecholamines. It functions as an oxidoreductase, with tetrahydropteridine as a cofactor, to convert L-tyrosine to L-dihydroxyphenylalanine (L-Dopa.).

NOTES

NOTES

8 Water Electrolyte and Acid Base Balance

1. Total body water in 70 kg man is: 60 % of body weight (42 L).
2. Major cation in intracellular fluid: Potassium.
3. Major cation of plasma: Sodium.
4. Major anion in intracellular fluid: Phosphate.
5. Major anion of extracelluler fluid: Chloride.
6. The osmolality of intra - and extracellular fluid is: 300 mosmoles/L.
7. The major regulatory factors of water and eletrolyte balance are: Hormones (aldosterone, ADH) and renin angiotensin system.
8. Acids are: Proton donors.
9. Bases are: Proton acceptors.
10. The acidity of a solution is measured by noting: H^+ ion concentration.
11. pH is defined as: -Log $[H^+]$.
12. The relationship between pH, pka, concentration of acid and conjugate base is expressed by Henderson - Hasselbalch equation: pH = Pka + log [Base] / [Acid].
13. Normal pH of blood is: 7.4 (7.35 to 7.45).
14. The solution which can resist changes in pH by addition of acid or alkali is: Buffer solution.
15. pk is defined as: pH at which an acid is half dissociated.
16. The major extracellular buffer is: Bicarbonate buffer system ($NaHCO_3$-H_2CO_3).
17. Normal pCO_2 of blood is: 40 mm Hg.
18. The major intracellular buffer is: Phosphate buffer (K_2HPO_4/ KH_2 PO_4).
19. Buffering capacity of protein depends on the: pka value of ionizable side chains.
20. The major mechanisms by which the kidney acts are:
    1. Excretion of H^+
    2. Reabsorption of filtered bicarbonate

3. Excretion of titrable acid
4. Excretion of NH_4^+.

21. In metabolic acidosis, there is increased excretion of: NH_4^+ ions.
22. In metabolic alkalosis, there is increased excretion of: HCO_3^-.

Acid-Base Abnormalities

Primary Disorder	Effect on PCO_2	Effect on HCO_3^-	Effect on pH	Compensation	Effect on PCO_2	Effect on HCO_3^-
Respiratory acidosis	Increase	–	decrease	Metabolic alkalosis	–	Increase
Respiratroy alkalosis	decrease	–	Increase	Metabolic acidosis	–	decrease
Metabolic acidosis	–	decrease	decrease	Respiratory alkalosis	decrease	–
Metabolic alkalosis	–	Increase	Increase	Respiratory acidosis	Increase	–

SOLVED QUESTIONS

Q.1. The buffering capacity of a buffer is maximum at pH equal to: **(AIPGME 2003)**

1. 0.5 pka
2. pka
3. pka+1
4. 2 pka.

Ans. **2**

Buffers are the substances that resist change in pH when an acid or base is added into the medium. The buffers are solutions of either weak acids or weak bases with their salt. At pka, the substance is 50 % ionized thus acts as effective buffer pH of 0.5 pka means pH< pka that is at an acidic pH the capacity of the buffer to resist change when an acid is added is greatly reduced pka+1 is alkaline pH and at an alkaline pH the capacity of the buffer to resist change when an alkali is added is greatly reduced .

Q.2. A buffer that is most effective at a pH of about 4.5 is:

1. Acetate
2. Bicarbonate
3. Phosphate
4. Tris buffer

Ans. **3**

Due to the Na $\longrightarrow$ H^+ exchange occurring at the renal tubular cell border, the $Na_2H\ PO_4$ is converted to $Na\ H_2\ PO_4$. The acid and basic phosphate pair is considered as the urinary buffer . The maximum limit of acidification is pH 4.5.

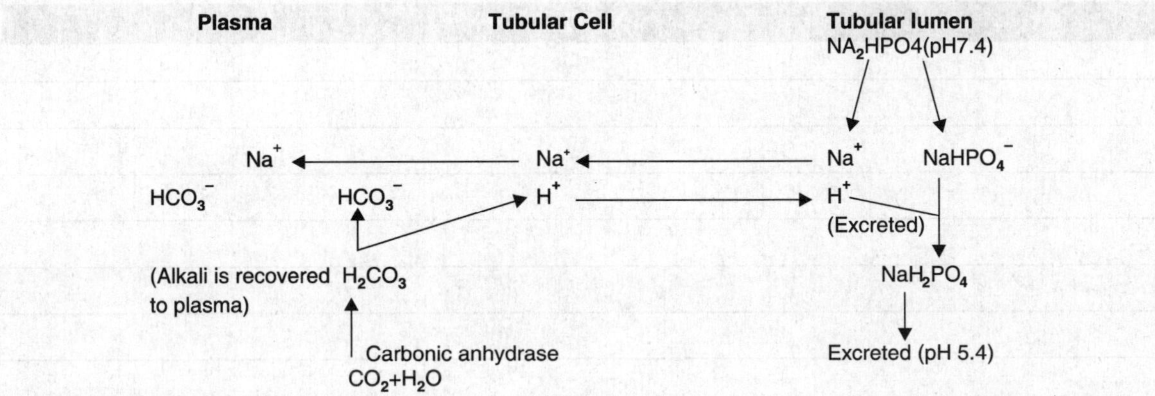

Q.3. In a solution the concentration of hydrogen ion [H^+] is 1´10^{-6} moles/litre. The pH of the solution will be: (AIIMS May 2006)

1. Three.
2. Six.
3. Nine.
4. Twelve.

Ans. **2**

$$PH = -\log [H^+]$$
$$= -\log [10^{-6}]$$
$$= 6$$

A low pH implies acidic solution and high pH implies basic solution. The strength of weak acid is expressed by pKa, the negative log of the acid dissociation constant. Strong acids have low pKa values and weak acids have high pKa values.

NOTES

9 Electron Transport Chain and Oxidative Phosphorylation

1. The energy changes during biochemical processes is known as: Bioenergetics.
2. A portion of the total energy change in a system that is available for doing work: Free energy.
3. Negative ΔG indicates that the reaction is: Spontaneous and exothermic.
4. Positive ΔG indicates that the reaction is: Endothermic.
5. Enzymes involved in biological oxidation are collectively called: Oxidoreductases.
6. Coenzymes for dehydrogenases are: NAD, NADP, or FAD or FMN.
7. Monooxygenases (cytochrome P_{450}) are involved in: Drug metabolism and steroid biosynthesis
8. The enzymes of the electron transport chain are embeded in the: Inner mitochondrial membrane.
9. Components of respiratory chain are arranged in order of: Increasing redox potential.
10. The inhibitors of complex - I are: Retenone, barbiturates, piericidin A.
11. The inhibitors of complex II is: Carboxin.
12. The mobile components of the respiratory chain: Coenzyme Q, cytochrome C.
13. The inhibitors of complex III are: Antimycin A, British Anti Lewisite.
14. The inhibitors of complex IV are: Cyanide, azide, Co, H_2S.
15. Transport of electrons through the ETC is: Exergonic process.
16. Oxidative phosphorylation is: Coupling of oxidation with phosphorylation.
17. For NAD^+ and FAD P:O ratio is approximately: 3 : 1 and 2 : 1.
18. The most accepted theory of oxidative phosphorylation is: Chemiosmotic theory.
19. The compounds which disrupt the coupling of oxidation with phosphorylation are: Uncouplers.
20. Uncoupling of oxidative phosphorylation causes: Oxidation to proceed but the energy is dissipated as heat.
21. The inhibitors of oxidative phosphorylation are: Atractyloside, oligomycin.
22. Physiological uncouplers are: Thyroxine, long chain fatty acids, bilirubin.
23. The other uncouplers include: 2, 4 - Dinitrophenol, dicumarol, dinitrocresol.

SOLVED QUESTIONS

Q.1. Cellular oxidation is inhibited by: **(AIPGME 2001)**

1. **Cyanide**
2. **Carbon dioxide**
3. **Chocolate**
4. **Carbonated beverages.**

Ans: 1

Cyanide inhibits cytochrome oxidase complex of respiratory chain. Cyanide binds with the heme of cytochrome oxidase and thus inhibits the terminal transfer of electrons to oxygen causing inhibition of cellular oxidation.

Q.2. In oxidative phosphorylation, the ATP production and respiratory chain are linked by: **(AIPGME 2002)**

1. **Chemical methods**
2. **Physical methods**
3. **Chemiosmotic methods**
4. **Conformational changes.**

Ans: 3

Chemiosmotic hypothesis proposed by Mitchell gives the link between ATP production and respiratory chain. It explains how the free energy generated by the electron transport in the electron transport chain is used to produce ATP from ADP and Pi. Electron transport is coupled with proton transport across inner mitochondrial membrane and the proton gradient generated is responsible for ATP synthesis.

Q.3. Spontaneous chemical reaction means free energy change is:

1. **Positive**
2. **Negative**
3. **Zero**
4. **Infinity.**

Ans: 2

If ΔG ie.free energy change is negative, the reaction proceeds spontaneously with loss of free energy, ie. it is exergonic. On the otherhand, if ΔG is positive, the reaction proceeds only if free energy can be gained, ie. it is endergonic.

Q.4. For which is cGMP second messenger:

1. **Thyroxine**
2. **Atrial natriuretic peptide**
3. **GH**
4. **Cortisone.**

Ans: **2**

The second messangers are the group of water soluble hormones that binds to the plasma membrane of the target cells to communicate with metabolic processes going on inside the cells by means of intermediary molecules called second messnagers. Whereas hormone itself is a first messanger. Only one hormone, atrial natriuretic factor (ANF), uses cGMP as its second messanger.

Q.5. Oxidative phosphorylation at the level of cytochrome oxidase is inhibited by:

1. **Carbon monoxide**
2. **Cyanide**
3. **Rofenone**
4. **Oligomycin.**

Ans: **1, 2**

Antimycin and dimercaprol inhibits the respiratory chain between cytochrome b and cytochrome c. The classic poisions H_2S, carbon monoxide, and cyanide inhibits cytochrome oxidase and can therefore totally arrest respiration.

The antibiotic oligomycin completely blocks oxidation and phosphorylation by acting on a step in phosphorylation.

Q.6. The specialized mammalian tissue/ organ in which fuel oxidation serves not to produce ATP but to generate heat is: (AIPGEE 2006)

1. **Adrenal gland.**
2. **Skeletal muscle.**
3. **Brown adipose tissue.**
4. **Heart.**

Ans: **3**

The process in which the oxidation serves not to produce ATP but to generate heat is known as thermogenesis. Brown adipose tissue is the site of this process. It is found in hibernating and new-born animals and is present in small quantity in humans.

The mitochondria of the brown adipose tissue are rich in electron carriers and are specialized to carry out an oxidation uncoupled from phosphorylation. This causes liberation of heat when fat is oxidized in the brown adipose tissue. The presence of active brown adipose tissue in certain individuals is believed to protect them becoming obese. The excess calories consumed by these people are burnt and liberated as heat, instead of being stored as fat.

Q.6. The electron flow in Cytochrome C oxidase can be blocked by: (AIIMS May 2006)

1. **Rotenone.**
2. **Antimycin A.**
3. **Cyanide.**
4. **Actinomycin**

Ans: 3

Many poisons inhibit the respiratory chain some of them are barbiturates such as amobarbital inhibit NAD linked dehydrogenases by blocking the transfer from FeS to Q. At sufficient dosage, they are fatal in vivo. Antimycin A and dimercaprol inhibit the respiratory chain between Cytochrome b and Cytochrome C. The classic poisons H_2S, carbon monoxide, and cyanide inhibit Cytochrome oxidase and can therefore totally arrest respiration.

NOTES

10

Heamoglobin

1. Hemoglobin is a: Conjugated protein (Chromoprotein).
2. Prosthetic group of hemoglobin is: Heme.
3. Each RBC contain: 280 million hemoglobin molecules.
4. Iron in hemoglobin is in the from of: Ferrous ion.
5. Adult type of hemoglobin is: HbA ($\alpha_2\beta_2$).
6. Fetal hemoglobin is: HbF ($\alpha_2\beta_2$).
7. The interaction between the subunits of Hb is by:
   (a) Noncovalent bonds like vander waal's forces and hydrogen bonds.
   (b) Intra and intersubunit salt bonds.
8. The form of Hb molecule in which 2,3, BPG enters the Hb molecule is: T-form.
9. The oxygen-binding curve for hemoglobin is: Sigmoidal.
10. High pCO_2 and low pH shifts the oxygen dissociation curve to: Right.
11. The oxygenation of Hb in the lungs and deoxygenation at the tissues under the effect of pH and pCO_2 is referred as: Bohr effect.
12. The buffering capacity of Hb is due to presence of amino acid.: Histidine.
13. Heme iron is oxidised to ferric form in: Methaemoglobinemia.
14. In patients with diabetes mellitus the derivative of Hb measured is: Glycosylated Hb.
15. Hemoglobin chesapeake is found in: Polycythemia.
16. Hemoglobin that do not produce any clinical symptoms: Hb P, Q, N, J.
17. Type of mutation in sickle cell anemia is: Base substitution (point mutation).
18. In sickle cell anemia, codon for glutamic acid (GAG) change to: Valine (GUG).
19. Polymerization of sickle cell hemoglobin occurs in: T-form (deoxygenated form).
20. In thalassemia the defect is in: Gene function but no abnormality in the polypeptide chains (i.e. amino acid sequence in polypeptide chain is normal but decreased or total absence of either α or β chains).

21. In porphyrine molecule, four pyrrole rings are linked by: α-Methenyl bridges.
22. Molecular weight of hemoglobin is: 64,500.
23. Molecular weight of myoglobin is: 17,000
24. The shape of oxygen saturation curve in case of myoglobin is: Hyperbolic.
25. All porphyrins have an absorption band near 400 nm, called: Soret band.
26. Heme biosynthesis occurs in most mammalian cells, except: RBC's.
27. Synthesis of heme occurs in: Mitochondria (upto ALA formation) and cytosol (from ALA to protoporphyrinogen II).
28. The immediate precursor is: Protoporphyrin IX.
29. The substrates for heme synthesis are: Succinyl CoA and glycine.
30. Rate limiting step in heme biosynthesis is: δ- Aminolevulinic acid synthetase.
31. The regulation of δ-ALA synthase is by: Feed back regulation.
32. A group of inborn errors of metabolism associated with the biosynthesis of heme are: Porphyrias.
33. All porphyrias are transmitted as autosomal dominant disorders except: Congenital erythropoietic porphyrias.
34. Loss of free Hb in kidney is prevented by: Haptoglobin.
35. The end products of heme catabolism are: Bile pigments.
36. Total hemoglobin in the body is about: 750 g.
37. Daily turnover rate is around: 6 g.
38. The porphyrin portion of heme is degraded in: R-E system of cells.
39. The by product of heme catabolism is: Carbon monoxide.
40. One gm of Hb produces: 35 mg of bilirubin.
41. Heme is degraded primarily by a microsomal enzyme system: Heme oxygenase.
42. The water insoluble bilirubin produced immediately after heme catabolism is: Unconjugated bilirubin.
43. Conjugation of bilirubin occurs in: Hepatocytes.
44. In plasma, unconjugated bilirubin is carried in a bound form with: Albumin.
45. Absorption of urobilinogen in intestine occurs at: Terminal ileum and large intesine.
46. In conjugated hyperbilirubinemia bilirubin occurs in: Smooth ER of hepatocytes, kidney, intestine.
47. In hyperbilirubinaemia blood bilirubin level exceeds: 1mg/dl.
48. Kernicterus occurs due to: Unconjugated bilirubin (> 20 mg/dl).
49. Jaundice appears when bilirubin concentration in blood becomes: 2-2.5 mg/dl.

SOLVED QUESTIONS

Q.1. In hemoglobin Iron is bound to: **(AIPGME 1995)**

1. Histidine

2. Leucine

3. **Isoleucine**
4. **Valine.**

Ans. 1

In hemoglobin iron remains in the ferrous state. It has 6 valencies. The iron is linked to the pyrrole nitrogen by 4 coordinate valency bonds. The fifth linkage is with the imidazole nitrogen of the proximal histidine (87th residue in alpha chain). In oxy-Hb, the 6th bond is with O_2 while in deoxy-Hb, a water molecule is present.

Q.2. Decreased glycolytic activity impairs oxygen transport by hemoglobin due to: (AIPGME 2003)

1. **Reduced energy production**
2. **Decreased production of 2,3- bisphosphoglycerate**
3. **Reduced synthesis of hemoglobin**
4. **Low levels of oxygen.**

Ans. 2

In the erythrocytes, the glycerophosphate kinase reaction of glycolysis is bypassed,. Bisphosphoglycerate mutase converts 1,3 bisphosphoglycerate to 2,3 bisphosphoglycerate (2,3 – BPG). The 2,3 –BPG has a high affinity for Hb. When it combines with Hb reduces the affinity towards oxygen. So in presene of 2,3 –BPG, oxy –Hb will unload oxygen more easily in tissues. But if glycolytic activity is decreased then 2,3 –BPG levels will deplete which impairs unload of oxygen in tissues.

Q.3. Porphobilinogen in urine produces pink colour with: (AIPGME 2003)

1. **Fouchet's reagent**
2. **Benedict's reagent**
3. **Sodium nitroprusside**
4. **Ehrlich's aldehyde reagent.**

Ans. 4

With Ehrlich's reagent porphobilinogen forms a red aldehyde compound which is insoluble in chloroform. Red colour after second extraction with chloroform means a positive test for porphobilinogen and highly suggestive of acute intermittent Porphyria.

Q.4. Which of the following can be a homologous substitution for valine in hemoglobin?

1. **Isoleucine**
2. **Glutamic acid**
3. **Phenylalanine**
4. **Lysine.**

Ans. 2

If valine at position 67 of the Beta – chain of Hb A molecule is replaced by glutamate it would result in Hb – Milwaukee which is functionally similar to Hb –A. So there is no change in the function of the Hb – molecule.

Q.5. Bilirubin is absent in urine because it is: (AIIMS 1999)

1. **Distributed in the body fat**
2. **Conjugated with glucuronide**
3. **Not filterable**
4. **Lipophilic.**

Ans. **4**

The uncojugated bilirubin is lipophilic so it cannot be excreted in urine.

Q.6. Which moiety of hemoglobin molecule binds 2,3- DPG at pH 7.0: (AIIMS JUNE 2000)

1. **Amino terminal**
2. **Carboxylic terminal**
3. **Sulfhydryl terminal**
4. **Alcoholic terminal.**

Ans. **1**

The hemoglobin tetramer binds one molecule of 2,3 – DPG in the central cavity formed by its four subunits. The space in the central cavity is sufficiently wide to accommodate BPG only when hemoglobin is in the T state . BPG forms salt bridges with the amino terminal amino groups of both β chains via val NA1 and with Lys EF_6 and His H21. Thus ,BPG stabilises deoxygenated (T state) Hb by forming additional salt bridges.

Q.7. True regarding conversion of deoxyhemoglobin to oxyhemoglobin is: (AIIMS MAY 2002)

1. **Binding of O_2 causes release of H^+**
2. **One mole of deoxyhemoglobin binds two moles of 2,3 –DPG**
3. **pH of blood has no effect on the binding of O_2**
4. **Binding of O_2 causes increased binding of 2,3-DPG.**

Ans. **1**

Hemoglobin performs two major functions in the body

1. Transport of O_2 from lungs to peripheral tissues
2. Transport of CO_2 and protons (H^+) from the peripheral tissues to the lungs.

At the tissue level oxy-Hb takes up a proton and release O_2 in the tissues. In lungs binding of O_2 to deoxy-Hb releases protons (H^+). The influence of pH and pCO_2 to facilitate oxygenation of Hb in the lungs and deoxygenation at the tissues is known as Bohr effect. One molecule of 2,3 – DPG binds with one molecule of deoxy Hb.2,3–DPG binds to deoxygenated (T) form of hemoglobin. Binding of 2,3–DPG with hemoglobin decreases binding with O_2 . Thus binding of 2,3 – DPG with

Hb favours release of O_2 to the tissues. In the tissues, pH is low due to the formation of metabolic acids. Then the affinity of Hb for O_2 is decreased (oxygen dissociation curve is shifted to the right) and so more O_2 is released to the tissues. In the lungs, opposite reaction is found. Thus pH affects O_2 binding with Hb.

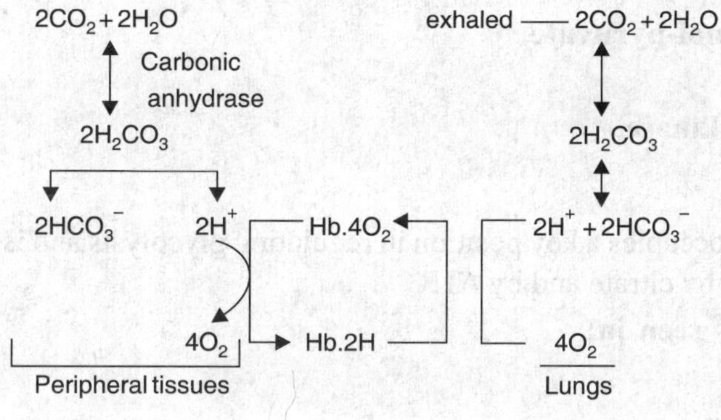

Q.8. Fluroacetate inhibits:

1. **Citrate synthetase**
2. **Aconitase**
3. **Succinic dehydrogenase**
4. **Alphaketoglutarate dehydrogenase.**

Ans. 2

Fluoroacetate is toxic because fluoroacetyl COA condenses with oxaloacetae to form fluorocitrate which inhibits aconitase, causing citrate to accumulate.

Q.9. All of the following factors are produced by hepatocytes except:

1. **Fibrinogen**
2. **Prothrombin**
3. **Von Willebrand factor**
4. **Factor VIII.**

Ans. 3

Von willebrand factor is a glycoprotein, secreted by endothelial cells into the plasma.

Q.10. Tyrosinemia type II is due to the deficiency of:

1. **Tyrosine aminotransferase**
2. **Fenanyl acetoacetyl hydrolase**
3. **Tyrosine hydroxylase**
4. **Tyrosinase.**

Ans. **1**

Tyrosinemia type II (Richner-hanhart syndrome) is caused due to the defect in the enzyme tyrosine aminotransferase which blocks the conversion of tyrosine to hydroxyphenyl pyruvate.

Q.11. Allosteric inhibition with ATP affects:

1. **Phosphofructokinase**
2. **Phosphoenol-pyruvate**
3. **G-6PD**
4. **Pyruvate kinase.**

Ans. **1**

Phosphofructokinase occupies a key position in regulating glycolysis and is also subject to feedback control. It is inhibited by citrate and by ATP.

Q.12. Triple helix is seen in:

1. **Collagen**
2. **Fibrinogen**
3. **Histones**
4. **Serum amylase.**

Ans. **1**

Collagen has a triple helix structure. A collagen triple helix has 3.3 residues per turn and rise per residence nearly twice that of an α -helix. The R groups of each polypeptide strand of the triple helix pack so closely that in order to fit, one must be glycine. So that every third residue in the collagen is glycine.

Q.13. Histamine is produced by:

1. **Oxidation**
2. **Reduction**
3. **Deamination**
4. **Decarboxylation.**

Ans. **4**

Histamine is formed from histidine by a decarboxylation catalyzed by L-amino acid decarboxylase.

Q.14. Lactate is transported from muscle to liver because:

1. **Liver has mitochondria**
2. **Lactate is stored in liver**
3. **Liver has glucose-6-phosphatase**
4. **Lactate is oxidized in liver.**

Ans. **3**

Lactate, formed by glycolysis in skeletal muscles and erythrocytes is transported to the liver and kidney where it reforms glucose via glucose-6-phosphate. This process is known as cori cycle or lactic acid cycle.

Q.15. Porphyrin is formed by joining together four pyrrole rings by means of ...... bridges:

1. **Hydrogen**
2. **Hydroxy**
3. **Phosphate**
4. **Methylene.**

Ans. 4

Uroporphyrinogens have the pyrrole ring connected by methylene bridges (-CH_2-) which do not form a conjugate ring system.

Q.16. What is the average number of high energy bonds required for the synthesis of 1 peptide bond?

1. **1**
2. **2**
3. **3**
4. **4.**

Ans. 4

The energy required for the formation of one peptide bond include the equivalent of the hydrolysis of two ATP molecules to ADP and of two GTP molecules to GDP or the hydrolysis of four high-energy phosphate bonds.

Q.17. The rate limiting enzyme in bile salt synthesis is:

1. **HMG-Co-A reductase**
2. **Decarboxylase**
3. **HMG-CoA synthetase**
4. **7-Alfa hydroxylase**

Ans. 4

The 7 α- hydroxylation of cholesterol is the first and principal regulatory step in the biosynthesis of bile acids catalyzed by 7 α- hydroxylase, a microsomal enzyme.

Q.18. Bile acids are formed from:

1. **Cholesterol**
2. **Amino acids**
3. **Bilirubin**
4. **Lipoproteins.**

Ans. 1

Bile acids are synthesized in liver from cholesterol

Q.19. Patients having obstructive jaundice do not excrete this at all in urine:

1. **Bilirubin**
2. **Glycocholate**
3. **Urobilinogen**
4. **Urate.**

Ans. 3

Normally, there are mere traces of urobilinogen in the urine. In complete obstruction of the bile duct, no urobilinogen is found in the urine, since bilirubin has no access to the intestine, where it can be converted to urobilinogen. In this case, the presence of bilirubin (conjugated) in the urine without urobilinogen suggests obstructive jaundice, either intrahepatic or post hepatic.

Q.20. There are more than three hundred variants of human hemoglobin gene. Among these only a few are fatal. Hence, the most important factor to be conserved in a protein for its function is the: (AIPGEE 2006)

1. **Amino acid sequence.**
2. **Ligand binding residues.**
3. **Structure.**
4. **Environment.**

Ans. 2

A molecule bound reversibly by a protein is called a 'ligand'. A ligand binds at a site on the protein called the 'binding site', which is complementary to ligand in size, charge and hydrophobic or hydrophilic character. As long as the ligand binding residues are preserved to allow interaction between the ligand and the binding sites the function will essentially be preserved.

11

Genetics

Chemistry of Nucleotides, Nucleosides and Nucleic Acids

1. Nucleotides are precursors of: Nucleic acids, DNA and RNA.
2. A nucleotide is made up of: Nitrogenous base + pentose sugar + phosphate group.
3. Nucleoside is: Pentose sugar + nitrogenous base.
4. Nitrogenous bases present in nucleotides are: Purines and pyrimidines.
5. Egs. of purine bases are: Adenine, guanine, hypoxanthine.
6. Eg. of pyrimidine bases are: Cytosine, thymine, uracil.
7. Adenine is: 6-amino purine (NH_2 group present at 6th position).
8. Guanine is**:** 2-amino, 6-oxy purine (NH_2 group is at 2nd position and O group at 6th position).
9. Minor bases which are present in small amounts in nucleic acids are**:** Hypoxanthine (6-oxopurine), xanthine (2, 6,-di-oxopurine).
10. Some of the methylated purine bases: N-methyl adenine, 5 methyl - cytosine,$N^5 N^6$- dimethyl adenine), 7 - Methyl guanine.
11. 1,3 dimethyl derivative of xanthine is called: Theophylline, present in tea.
12. The nitrogen atom of purine or pyrimidine to which the (C_1) sugar is attached to from a nucleoside are: N_9 of a purine and N_1 of pyrimidine.
13. The phosphate group in a nucleotide is generally attached to: 3' or 5' carbon of the sugar.
14. Nucleotide molecules at physiological pH bear a**:** Negative charge.

Functions of Nucleotides

1. Nucleotides serve as monomer units for synthesis of DNA and RNA.
2. ATP provides energy, cAMP acts as 2nd messenger, PAPS acts as SO_4 donor, SAM acts as methyl donor, FMN, FAD, NAD, NADP, Co A act as coenzymes.
3. GTP provides energy, cGMP acts as second messenger.

4. CDP choline and CDP ethanolamine are used for phospholipid synthesis. CMP N-acetyl neuraminic acid is used for ganglioside synthesis.
5. UDP glucose is used for synthesis of glycogen.

CHEMISTRY OF NUCLEIC ACIDS

1. Many mononucleotides are joined to each other by phosphodiester bonds to form: Polynucleotide.
2. Two important polynucleotides are DNA and RNA which are the polymers of deoxy ribo nucleotides and ribonucleotides respectively.
3. The structure of double stranded DNA structure was first proposed by: Watson, Crick.
4. In a double stranded DNA molecule two strands of DNA are held together by: Hydrogen bonds (3 between G and C, 2 between A and T).
5. Always the two strands of DNA are: Complementary and antiparallel to each other.
6. Chargaffs rule where base pairing in DNA strands is A=T, G≡C: states that: The number of purines is equal to the number of pyrimidines.
7. The right handed double helical DNA has a pitch of: 3.4 nm per turn.
   The number of bases per turn: 10 base pairs
   The diameter or width of the helix: 1.9 - 2.0 nm.
8. The perdominant form of DNA under physiological conditions is: 'B' form and other forms are A, C, D, E, Z.
9. Denaturtion and separation of double stranded DNA by heat is called: Melting of DNA.
10. Regions of DNA that are more resistant to denaturation: G-C pair - containing regions.
11. DNA in mitochondria exists in the form of: Circular DNA.
12. Double stranded DNA wound over histones is called: Nucleosome.
13. Chromatin in the nucleus is made of: Double stranded DNA + Histones + Non histone proteins + RNA.
14. The basic amino acids found in high concentration in histones are: Lysine and arginine.
15. Number of base pairs of DNA in each haploid genome of human cell: 7 $X10^9$ base pairs.
16. Only about 10 % of the human DNA contain genes; The rest are silent areas.
17. The segments of the gene coding for proteins are called as: Exons (expressed regions) interspaced with stretches of silent areas called introns (intervening areas).
18. The unit of genetic expression is: Cistron.
19. Transcriptionally active and inactive chromatin are respectively called as: Euchromatin and heterochromatin.
20. Chromosomes in metaphase are: Transcriptionally inactive.
21. RNA differs from DNA:
    (i) It contains U, DNA has T
    (ii) It contains ribose

(iii) It is single stranded

(iv) It doesn't obey chargaff's rule.

22. Types of RNA found inside the cell are: Messenger (m) RNA, transfer (t)RNA, Ribosomal (r) RNA, hetero nuclear (hn) m RNA, small nuclear (Sn) RNA.
23. RNA having clover leaf like structure is: t-RNA.

METABOLISM OF NUCLEOTIDES AND NUCLEIC ACIDS.

1. Major pathway for biosynthesis of purines and pyrimidines is: De Novo synthesis (operates in cytoplasm).
2. Rate limiting enzyme in de novo purine biosynthesis: PRPP synthetase.
3. Sources for the synthesis of purine ring: CO_2 glycine, amide N of glutamine, methenyl THFA, formyl THFA and NH_2 group of aspartate.
4. Since human being can syntheisze the purine and pyrimidine bases de novo , they are called as: Prototrophs.
5. Pathway used for the biosynthesis of nucleotides from preformed purines and pyrimidines and their nudeosides is: Salvage pathway.
6. Salvage pathway operates in tissues like: RBC and brain where de novo pathway is not operating. This pathway economises intracellular energy expenditure as by de novo synthesis, one molecule of purine requires about 6 ATP for its synthesis.
7. Common sunbstrate for denovo synthesis pathway and salvage pathway is: PRPP.
8. The end product of purine nucleotide catabolism is: Uric acid (urate).
9. Rate limiting enzyme in uric acid synthesis is: Xanthine oxidase.
10. Xanthine oxidase is inhibited by the drug: Allopurinol.
11. The normal blood level of uric acid: Males-3-7 mg/.dl. Females- 2-5 mg /dl.
12. The most common abnormality of purine metabolism is: An elevation of uric acid level in blood: Hyperuricemia.
13. Hyperuricemia is seen in metabolic disorders of purine metabolism like: Gout, Lesch- Nyhan syndrome.
14. The enzymes defective in gout are: 5 - PRA transferase and PRPP synthetase (abnormal forms).
15. The biochemical defect in Lesch - Nyhan syndrome is deficiency of: Hypoxanthine guanine phosphoribosyl transferase (HGPR Tase).
16. Sources for synthesis of pyrimidine ring: Carbamoyl phosphate and aspartic acid.
17. The enzyme carbamoyl phosphate synthetase required for pyrimidine biosynthesis is persent in: Cytosol of cell.
18. The metabolic disorder associated with pyrimidine metabolism is: Orotic aciduria.
19. The deficient enzymes of orotic aciduria are: OPR Tase(Orotic phospho ribosyl transferase and OMP (orotidine monophosphate) decarboxylase.
20. Drugs precipitating orotic aciduria: Allopurinol and 6-Azauridine.

21. The first enzyme in pyrimidine de novo synthesis pathway, carbamoyl phosphate synthase II is inhibited by: UTP.
22. The type of DNA replication in eukaryotes is: Semiconservative.
23. DNA polymerase enzyme which synthesizes a new complementary strand DNA is located in: Nucleus.
24. Initiation of DNA synthesis requires priming by: Short length of RNA.
25. DNA synthesis is always in the direction: 5' to 3' in both strands.
26. The discontinuously synthesized and continuously polymerised strands of DNA are: Lagging strand and leading strand respectively.
27. DNA Fragments synthesized at the lagging strand are called: Okazaki fragments.
28. The gaps between new fragments of DNA are sealed by: DNA ligases.
29. The phase of cell cycle in which DNA synthesis occurs: S phase.
30. A unit of DNA that contains signal for initiation of DNA synthesis is: Replicon.
31. Supercoiling of DNA is mediated by: Topoisomerases and gyrases.
32. Eukaryotes have multiple sites of origin of DNA replication called as: Autonomous replicating sequences.
33. An auto somal recessive condition caused due to xerodema a defective nucleotide excision repair mechanism is: Xeroderma pigmentosum.
34. The end piece of the chromosome where strands connot be replicated is: Telomere.
35. The shortening of telomere end is prevented by: Telomerase.
36. Telomerases have been implicated in: Ageing process and cancers.
37. The most heterogeneous class of RNA is: m RNA.
38. The process of synthesis of RNA from DNA is: Transcription.
39. Transcription unit of DNA extends from promoter site to: Terminator site.
40. RNA is synthesized from DNA by: RNA polymerase.
41. The mRNA formed and released from the DNA template is known as: Primary transcript /hn RNA.
42. The post transcriptional modifications of primary transcript produces mature mRNA by: 7 methyl guanosine triphosphate capping at 5' end and poly adenylated tailing at 3` end.
43. Enzyme that synthesizes double stranded DNA complementary from single stranded RNA is called: Reverse transcriptase.
44. tRNA is transcribed by the enzyme: DNA dependent RNA polymerase III.
45. Transfer of amino acids from cytoplasm to the ribosomal protein synthesising machinery is done by: tRNA
46. The amino acids for protein synthesis are attached to the tRNA at the: Acceptor arm.
47. The tRNA has 5 arms: Acceptor anticodon, D, T Ψ C, variable.
48. mRNA is translated into protein with the help of: Ribosomes.
49. The two subunits of ribosomes are: Composed of RNA and protein.

50. Ribosome of eukaryotes is: 80s'.
51. Translation of codons of m RNA into amino acids is done by: tRNA.
52. The number of codons that code for specific amino acids: 61, Total = 64 (3 stop cadons).
53. Translation occurs in: Cytosol.
54. Post -translational modifications for forming active protein: Proteolytic cleavage and modifications of amino acids.
55. Carboxylation reactions (Eg. carboxylation of glutamate of prothrombin) are influenced by: Vitamin K
56. Hydroxylation of proline and lysine in collagen is with the help of: Vitamin C.
57. Correct spatial arrangement and prevention of wrong foldings of proteins is with the help of: Chaperons.
58. Chain terminating codons are: UAA, UAG, UGA.
59. Transition occurs when: A purine is replaced by a purine or a pyrimidine is replaced by pyrimidine.
60. The type of mutation where purine replaces pyrimidine or viceversa is: Transversion.
61. Exposure to U-V light causes: Formation of thymine dimers in DNA (T-Tdimer).
62. The binding of regulatory proteins to DNA is mediated by: Specific motifs (helix turn helix, zinc-finger and Leucine zipper).
63. A unit of gene experssion is: Operon.
64. Inducers of lac operon are: Allolactose and cAMP.
65. Programmed cell death is called: Apoptosis.

Genetic Engineering

1. The exchange of genetic information between two DNA segments is: Genetic recombination.
2. Enzyme that cut DNA at specific suquence are: Restriction endonucleases.
3. Different vectors used to introduce the human gene into bacteria are: Plasmids, bacteriophages and cosmids.
4. A vector carrying a foreign DNA is called: Chimeric DNA or hybrid DNA or recombinant DNA.
5. DNA libraries are: Genomic library and complementary DNA library.
6. Genomic library represents: Entire genome of an organism.
7. cDNA library represents: mRNA species in an organism.
8. The various blotting techniques are:

   Southern blotting for: Identifying DNA

   Northern blotting for: Identifying RNA

   Western blotting for: Analysis of proteins.
9. In vitro DNA amplification procedure is: Polymerase chain reaciton.
10. During PCR new DNA strands are synthesized by: Thermostable DNA polymerase (Taq Polymerase).

11. Uses of PCR:
   (i) Diagnosis of bacterial and viral diseases
   (ii) Medicolegal cases
   (iii) Diagnosis of genectic disorders
   (iv) Cancer detection
   (v) Paleontogical studies.

SOLVED QUESTIONS

Q.1. Which is not found in DNA? **(AIPGME 1994)**

1. Adenine
2. Thymine
3. Guanine
4. Uracil.

Ans. **4**

There are two types of nitrogen bases in DNA- purine and pyrimidine. Purine bases are – adenine, guanine, pyrimidine bases are – Cytosine, thymine.

Q.2. On complete hydrolysis, of DNA, we will get all of the following except: **(AIPGME 1994)**

1. Adenosine
2. Purine base
3. Phosphoric acid
4. Dexose pentose sugar.

Ans. **1**

Adenosine is a nucleoside, composed of adenine (a purine base) and ribose (pentose sugar). On complete hydrolysis, all the components of DNA are separated into individual nitrogen bases, phosphoric acid and pentose sugar. So a nucleoside (adenosine) would be separated by hydrolysis.

Q.4. Which form of DNA is predominantly seen? **(AIPGME 1994)**

1. A
2. C
3. B
4. Z.

Ans. **3**

The structure described by Watson and Crick (Right handed double helix) is denoted as the B form which is predominantly seen under physiological conditions.The A form is bulkier than B form and has more base pairs per turn. C,D, and E forms are seen under artificial conditions. A,B,C,D, and E, forms right handed helices; while the Z form is left hended. In Z form, the phosphodiester bridges form zigzag and hence the name.

Q.5. Thermo – stability in DNA is contributed mostly by: (AIPGME 1996)

1. **A=T**
2. **G≡C**
3. **molecular base**
4. **Parallel arrangement.**

Ans. 2

The two strands of DNA are held together by hydrogen bonds present between the nitrogen bases Between adenine and thymine two hydrogen bonds are present while between guanine and cytosine three hydrogen bonds are present. Thus G≡C base pair is more stable than A=T base pair. So thermo-stability in DNA is mostly because of G≡C base pairs.

Q.6. Okazaki fragments helps in: (AIPGME 1996)

1. **DNA replication**
2. **Translation**
3. **Protein synthesis**
4. **Transcription.**

Ans. 1

DNA polymerase III catalyses main replication. It adds deoxyribonucleotides in 5' → 3' direction , so new strand synthesis on 3' → 5' parent strand is continuous. While on 5' → 3' parent strand new strand is synthesized in a discontinuous manner. These short stretches of deoxy-ribonucleotides are added on primer RNA which are added by RNA primase. These small pieces of deoxy ribonucleotides attached to its own primer RNA are called okazaki fragments.

Q.7. Binding of proteins to DNA is regulated by: (AIPGME 1996)

1. **Copper**
2. **Zinc**
3. **Selenium**
4. **Nickel.**

Ans. 2

The specificity involved in the control of transcriptions requires that regulatory proteins bind with high affinity to the correct region of DNA. Three unique motifs-

(i) helix–turn – helix

(ii) zinc finger and

(iii) Leucine zipper- accounts for specific protein -DNA interactions.of 5S RNA transcription, requires zinc for activity. Each TF III A molecule contains 9 zinc ions.

Q.8. Which enzyme involved in translation is often referred to as 'Fidelity enzyme': (AIPGME 1997)

1. **DNA polymerase**
2. **RNA polymerase**
3. **Amino acyl-tRNA synthetase**
4. **Amino acyl reductase.**

Ans. **3**

Among the given choices aminoacyl–tRNA synthetase is the enzyme involved in translation. The enzyme activates the amino acids. The enzyme identifies the specific tRNA and transfers the aminoacyl group to the CCA 3' end of tRNA.The fidelity of translation resides in the specificity of the enzyme.The enzyme is highly selective in the recognition of both-the amino acid and the tRNA acceptor. DNA polymerase is the enzyme of DNA replication and RNA polymerase is the enzyme of transcription (RNA synthesis).

Q.9. Okazaki segments are required for: **(AIPGME 1998)**

1. **DNA synthesis**
2. **RNA synthesis**
3. **Protein synthesis**
4. **None of the above.**

Ans. **1**

Okazaki fragments are small pieces of deoxyribonucleotides attached to its own primer RNA. They are synthesized during DNA replication. Once they are generated, replication complex begins to remove RNA, primers, to fill in the gaps left by their removal with proper base paired deoxyribonucleotide and then to seal the fragments by DNA ligase.

Q.10. Translation occurs in: **(AIPGME 1999)**

1. **Ribosomes**
2. **Mitochondria**
3. **Nucleus**
4. **Cytoplasm.**

Ans. **1**

Site of protein synthesis is ribosome. mRNA attaches with small subunit of ribosome while large subunit has two sites-one for peptidyl-tRNA and another for amino acyl- tRNA specific proteins and rRNA molecules present in both the ribosomal subunits also help in translation.

Q.11. Gout is a disorder of: **(AIPGME 1999)**

1. **Purine metabolism**
2. **Pyrimidine metabolism**
3. **Oxalate metabolism**
4. **Protein metabolism.**

Ans. **1**

End product of purine catabolism in humans is uric acid.Excessive accumulation of uric acid crystals in the synovial fluid results in inflammation leading to gouty arthritis.Lack of control of the enzymes 5- phosphoribosyl amino transferase and PRPP synthase, deficiency of enzymes of salvage pathway are some reasons which will lead to excessive uric acid production.

Q.12. Aminoacyl tRNA is required fro all Except: **(AIPGME 2000)**

1. **Hydroxyprorline**
2. **Methionine**
3. **Cystine**
4. **Lysine.**

Ans. **1**

Methionine, cystine, lysine are all amino acids which are activated by aminoacyl t-RNA. First proline is introduced by amino acyl t-RNA into polypeptide chain and afterwards as a post translational modification, hydroxylation of proline occurs. So proline is hydroxylated to hydroxyproline after polypeptide chain synthesis.

Q.13. The primary defect in xeroderma pigmentosa is: **(AIPGME 2000)**

1. **Formation of thymidine dimers**
2. **Poly ADP ribose polymerase is defective**
3. **Exonuclease is defective**
4. **Formation of adenine dimers.**

Ans. **3**

In xeroderma pigmentosa defect lies in the nucleotide exision repair mechanism to remove T-T dimers. Thus a specific exonuclease is defective.

Q.14. Null mutation is: **(AIPGME 2000)**

1. **Mutation occurring in noncoding region**
2. **Mutation that does not change the amino acid or end product**
3. **Mutation that codes for a change in progeny without any chromosomal change**
4. **Mutation that leads to no functional gene product.**

Ans. **4**

Null mutation is the mutation that eliminates the gene function. As gene function is lost no functional gene product is produced .

Q.15. Triple bonds are found between which base pairs: **(AIPGME 2001)**

1. **A-T**
2. **C-G**
3. **A-G**
4. **C-T.**

Ans. **2**

Triple hydrogen bonds are present between guanine and cytosine:

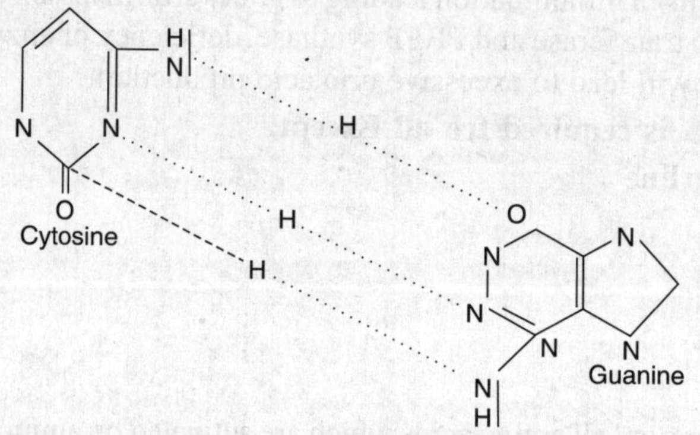

Q.16. Which of the following RNA has abnormal purine bases? (AIPGME 2001)

1. **tRNA**
2. **mRNA**
3. **rRNA**
4. **16S RNA.**

Ans. **1**

tRNA contain a significant proportion of unusual bases. These include dihydrouracil (DHU), pseudouridine (Ψ) and hypoxanthine. Many methylated bases are also present. The 5'- end often has a a phosphorylated guanosine. Thymine is present only in tRNA while thymine is absent in other RNA molecules.

Q.17. 'False' regarding gout is: (AIPGME 2002)

1. **Due to increased metabolism of pyrimidines**
2. **Due to increased metabolism of purines**
3. **Uric acid levels may not be elevated**
4. **Has a predilection for the great toe.**

Ans. **1**

Pyrimidine nucleotides are degraded to β- alanine and β-aminoisobutyrate which are highly soluble. So no clinical manifestations are observed.End product of purine catabolism in humans is uric acid. Excess of urate crystals get deposited in the synovial fluid resulting into gouty arthritis, Hyperuricemia is a necessary but not a sufficient pre-requisite for clinical features of gout.

Q.18. All the following can be used to detect mutation, except: (AIPGME 2002)

1. **Single strand conformational polymorphism**
2. **Ligase chain reaction**
3. **Polymerase chain reaction**
4. **DNA Sequencing.**

Ans. **3**

Single strand conformational polymorphism also called restrictions fragment length polymorphism. It is a technique in which restriction fragment markers that demonstrate tight linkage to a mutant phenotype. A change in DNA sequance may lead to a gain or loss of restriction enzyme recognition site resulting in different sized restriction fragments. These fragments are detected by southern blot analysis. Ligase chain reactions is used to seal the gap produced during DNA repair mechanism. DNA sequencing is based on constructing a complementary DNA copy of the molecule. Polymerase chain reaction involves in vitro DNA amplification producing millions of copies of particular DNA.

Q.19. The protein rich in basic amino acids, which functions in the packaging of DNA in chromosomes is: (AIPGME 2003)

1. **Histone**
2. **Collagen**
3. **Hyaluronic acid binding protein**
4. **Fibrinogen.**

Ans. **1**

Histones, present in DNA are basic in nature. They contain two basic amino acids lysine and arginine which are responsible for basic nature of histones.There are 5 classes of histones H_1, H_2A, H_2B, H_3 and H_4. The double strand wraps twice around a histone octamer formed by H_2A, H_2B, H_3 and H_4. This super- twisted helix is nucleosomes. H_1 histone is present at the site where DNA leaves the octamer. Supercoiled nucleosomes form chromatin fibres. Chromatin is further condensed to form chromosomes.

Q.20. Which of the following is not a post transcriptional modification of RNA? (AIPGME 2003)

1. **Splicing**
2. **5' Capping**
3. **3' Polyadenylation**
4. **Glycosylation.**

Ans. **4**

Glycosylation is post translational modification of protein for the formation of glycoprotein. After transcriptions, primary transcript produced undergoes extensive editing to become the mature mRNA. These modifications are endonuclease cleavage, poly - A tailing at 3' end, 5'capping, methylation, removal of introns and connection of exons.

Q.21. Shine-Dalgarno sequence in bacterial mRNA is near: (AIPGME 2004)

1. **AUG codon**
2. **UAA codon**
3. **UAG codon**
4. **UGA codon.**

Ans. **1**

Shine – Dalgarno sequence is a purine rich sequence which is similar to the sequence AGGAGGU. This sequence base pairs with a pyrimidine sequence in the 16s r RNA present is 30 s ribosomal sub unit. Shine- Dalgarno sequence lies within 10 nucleotides of the initiator codon. It places the initiator codon in the appropriate position in the 30S subunit to bind with initiator tRNA.

Q.22. RNA polymerase does not require: **(AIPGME 2004)**

1. **Template (dsDNA)**
2. **Activated precursors (ATP,GTP, UTP, CTP)**
3. **Divalent metal ions (Mg^{++} $Mn2^{+}$)**
4. **Primer.**

Ans. **4**

RNA polymerase is an enzyme of transcription RNA molecule is synthesized on one strand of DNA (template strand.) It needs the substrates ATP, CTP, UTP and GTP. RNA Polymerase dose not require RNA primers for RNA synthesis. RNA chain is synthesized in 5′ — 3′ direction on 5′ — 3′ template DNA strand.

Q.23. A segments of eukaryotic gene that is not represented in the mature mRNA, is known as: **(AIPGME 2004)**

1. **Intron**
2. **Exon**
3. **Plasmid**
4. **TATA Box.**

Ans. **1**

The primary transcripts are very long. They contain coding regions (exons) interspersed with non - coding regions (introns). These intron sequences are cleaved and the exons are spliced together to form the mature mRNA.

Q.24. Xeroderma pigmentosum is produced as a result of a defect in: **(AIPGME 2004)**

1. **DNA polymerase III**
2. **DNA polymerase I**
3. **DNA exonuclease**
4. **DNA ligase**

Ans. **3**

Explanation same as Q . 13.

Q.25. What is meant by melting of double stranded DNA? **(AIIMS JUNE 1998)**

1. **Splitting of double strands into single strand**
2. **Splitting of DNA into fragments**

3. Formation of triple helix
4. Separation of bases.

Ans. 1

Melting involves splitting of hydrogen bonds present between the nitrogen bases . As these bonds break double stranded DNA split into single strands.

Q.26. For measurement of long DNA molecules (50-100kb) following is used:
(AIIMS DEC 1998)

1. Chromsome walking
2. Nitch
3. RFLP
4. SSLP.

Ans. 1

In chromosome walking a fragment representing one end of a long piece of DNA is used to isolate another that overlaps but extends the first. The direction of extension is determined by restriction mapping and the procedure repeated sequentially until the desired sequence is obtained

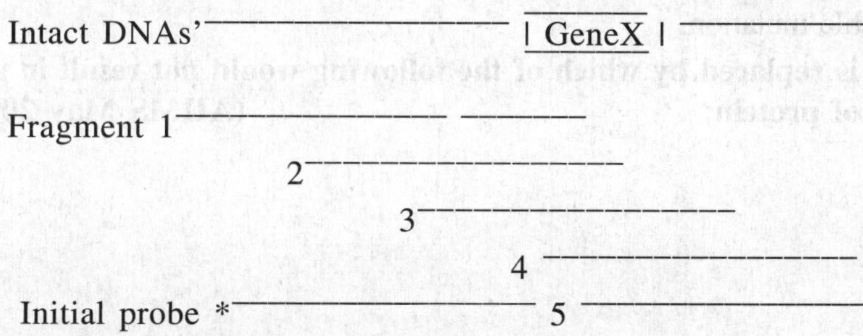

Q.27. Which of these is a conservative mutator?

1. Glutamic acid – glutamine
2. Histidine – glycine
3. Alanine – leucine
4. Arginine – aspartic acid.

Ans. 1

Q.28. Amber codon refers to: **(AIIMS MAY 2001)**

1. Mutant codon
2. Stop codon
3. Initiating codon
4. Condon for more than one amino acids.

Ans. 2

Amber codon is terminator codon or stop codon. It is a codon which do not code for any particular amino acids

UAA - Amber codon

UAG - Ochre codon

UGA - Opel codon.

Q.29. A mutation in the codon which causes a change in the coded amino acid is known as: (AIIMS MAY 2001)

1. Mitogenesis
2. Somatic mutation
3. Missense mutation
4. Recombination.

Ans. 3

Missense mutation causes substitution of amino acid. Thus missense mutation in codon changes the coded amino acid missense mutations are of three types:

(i) Missense but acceptable mutation
(ii) Missense: partially acceptable mutation
(iii) Missense: Unacceptable mutation.

Q.30. In a mutation if valine is replaced by which of the following would not result in any change in the function of protein: (AIIMS May 2002)

1. Proline
2. Leucine
3. Glycine
4. Aspartic acid.

Ans. 4

In a mutation if valine at positon 67 of beta chain of normal Hb A is replaced by aspartic acid it would not affect the function of Hb. GUU codon which codes for valine after point mutation changes to GAU which code for aspartate and this Hb is then called Hb Bristol. Similarly replacement of valine by following amino acid would not affect the function of Hb.

Valine (GUU) ⟶ Alanine (GCU): Hb sydney

Valine (GUU) ⟶ Glutamate (GAA); Hb Milwaukee

Valine (GUU) ⟶ Aspartate (GAU)): H b Bristol

This is applicable only for hemoglobin and not for other proteins.

Q.31. In a DNA, the coding region reads 5'-CGT –3'. This would code in the RNA as: (AIIMS May 2002)

1. 5'-CGU-3'
2. 5' GCA 3'
3. 5'-ACG –3'

4. 5'-UGC –3'.

Ans. **1**

During transcription RNA is synthesized on a template strand (noncoding strand) in 5'-3' direction. Another strand on DNA is called coding strand because its base sequence is similar with the base sequence present on mRNA (codons); only difference is at places where there is thymine in coding strand uracil is present on RNA molecule otherwise rest of the sequence is same. Hence, if the sequence on coding strand is 5'-CGT -3' then on RNA sequence will be the same 5'-CGU-3' or if the sequence on coding strand is 5'-CGT-3' then on template strand the sequence is 3'GCA-5' and and on mRNA it will be 5'-CGU-3'

Q.32. At the physiological pH the DNA molecules are: **(AIIMS NOV 2002)**

1. Positively charged

2. Negatively charged

3. Neutral

4. Amphipathic.

Ans. **2**

Because of phosphoric acid = p = at physiological pH the DNA molecules are negatively charged.

Q.33. Excessive ultraviolet (uv) radiation is harmful to life. The damage caused to the biological systems by ultraviolet radiation is by: **(AIIMS May 2004)**

1. Inhibition of DNA synthesis

2. Formation of thymidine dimers

3. Ionization

4. DNA fragmentation.

Ans. **2**

Pyrimidine dimers (thymidine dimers) are produced by photons, particularly u.v/ light repair is effected by reversing this damage by DNA photolyases, using $FADH_2$ and THFA as coenzymes.

Q.34. Restriction endonuclease is:

1. Break single stranded DNA

2. Break double stranded DNA

3. Break peptide chain

4. Break RNA.

Ans. **2**

Restriction endonuleases have a specific recognition site. Each enzyme recognizes and cleaves a specific double stranded DNA sequence. Restriction enzymes cut DNA of any source into short pieces in a sequence specific manner.

Q.35. DNA restriction is done by the following method:

1. **Paper chromatography**
2. **Electrophoresis agargel method**
3. **Spectrophotometer**
4. **Spectrometry.**

Ans. **2**

DNA framents obtained by the action of restriction endonucleases are electrophoresed on agar / agarose gel DNA being negatively charged , migrates towards the anode. The agar/ agarose support is used to separate different types of protein mixtures. Good separation is obtained with agar/ agarose gel electrophoresis.

Q.36. Thermostability of DNA is provided by:

1. **G ≡ C bonds**
2. **A = T pairing**
3. **N-glycosolic bond**
4. **Antiparallel arrangement.**

Ans. **1**

DNA rich in G ≡ C pairs, which have three hydrogen bonds melts at a higher temperature than that rich in A = T pairs, which have two hydrogen bonds. A ten fold increase of monovalent cation concentration increases the T_m by 166^0 C. This allows the strands of DNA or DNA-RNA hybrids to be separated at much lower termperatures and minimizes the phosphodiester bond breakage that occurs at high temperatures.

Q.37. True about polymerase chain reaction is:

1. **Enzymatic DNA amplification**
2. **Recombiant DNA amplification**
3. **Separation of protein fragments in serum**
4. **None**

Ans. **1**

The polymerase chain reaction is a method of amplifying a target sequence of DNA. Two oligonucleotide primers that hybridize to complementary sequences on opposite strands of DNA are used. Along with primer, substrates ATP,CTP, TTP, and GTP as well as the enzyme DNA polymerase is added to the medium. Thus it is just the enzymatic DNA amplification.

Q.38. DNA fragments formed by the action of restriction endonucleases. are separated by: (AIPGME 2000)

1. **Gel electrophoresis**
2. **Agarose gel electrophoresis**
3. **Paper chromatography**

4. High pressure liquid chromatography.

Ans. 2

Explanation same as Q.35

Q.39. Restriction fragment length polymorphism is used for: **(AIPGME 2003)**

1. Analysis of chromosome structure

2. DNA estimation

3. Synthesis of nucleic acid

4. Detecting proteins in a cell.

Ans. 1

The differences in DNA sequence can result in variations of restriction sites and thus in the length of restriction fragments. An inherited difference in the pattern of restriction is known as restriction fragment length polymorphism. RFLP map is useful in the human genome sequencing project. RFLPs can be used to establish linkage groups, which in turn, by the process of chromosome walking , will define the disease locus. RFLPs are inherited.

Q.40. An enzyme that makes a double stranded DNA copy from a single stranded RNA template molecule is known as: **(AIPGME 2004)**

1. DNA polymerase

2. RNA polymerase

3. Reverse transcriptase

4. Phosphokinase.

Ans. 3

A class of enzymes capable of synthesizing a single stranded and then a double stranded DNA molecule from a single stranded RNA template. This RNA – dependent DNA polymerase is called reverse transcriptase . Retroviruses have this class of enzymes.

Q.41. Northern blot test is used for:

1. DNA analysis

2. RNA analysis

3. Analysis of proteins

4. Enzyme analysis.

Ans. 2

The northern blot is used to demonstrate specific RNA. The total RNA is isolated from the cell, electrophoresed and then blotted on to a membrane. This is then probed with radioactive cDNA. There will be RNA –DNA hybridization , if the specific RNA (complementary to DNA probe) is present in the cell. For DNA analysis southern blot technique is used western blot analysis is used to identify the proteins.

Q.42. An enzyme that makes a double stranded DNA copy from a single stranded RNA template molecule is known as:

1. **DNA polymerase**
2. **RNA polymerase**
3. **Reverse transcriptase**
4. **Phosphokinase.**

Ans. 3

Q.43. The codon of which amino acid is also an initiating codon for proteins:

1. **Leucine**
2. **Isoleucine**
3. **Methionine**
4. **Lysine.**

Ans. 3

The codon of methionine is AUG which is the initiation codon for translation mechanism of all proteins.

Q.44. The diploid number of chromosomes is perpetuated in somatic cells by a process of:

1. **Meiosis**
2. **Mitosis**
3. **Amitosis**
4. **Cytokinesis**

Ans. 2

Mitosis is the process in which the number of chromosomes in daughter cells remains the same as the parent cell. So the diploid number of chromosomes is perpetuated is somatic cells by a process of mitosis. Meiosis reduces the number of chromosomes to half in daughter cells. Meiosis occurs during gamete formation.

Q.45. A genetic aberration resulting in enzyme deficiencies and causing severe immune deficiency states in the patient is due to absence of which enzyme:

1. **Hypoxanthine guanine phosphoribosyl transferase**
2. **Adenosine deaminase**
3. **Xanthine oxidase**
4. **Guanine deaminase.**

Ans. 2

Adenosine deaminase deficiency is associated with severe immuno deficiency where both T and B cells are deficient. It is an inherited autosomal recessive disease. Accumulation of deoxyribonucleotides would inhibit further production of precursors of DNA synthesis especially d CTP.

Q.46. In sickle cell anaemia, the defect can be explained as having arisen from:

1. **A base insertion in DNA**
2. **A base deletion in DNA**
3. **A base substitution in DNA**
4. **None of the above.**

Ans. 3

In the DNA molecule glutamic acid, the normal amino acid in position 6 of the β -chain, has been replaced by valine. The corresponding single nucleotide change within the codon would be GAA or GAG of glutamic acid to GUA or GUG of valine. Clearly, this missense mutation hinders normal functions and results in sickle cell anemia when the mutant gene is present in the homozygous state.

Q.47. DNA double helix is bound by:

1. **Covalent bond**
2. **Hydrogen bond**
3. **Disulfide linkage**
4. **Vander wal forces.**

Ans. 2

The two strands of the DNA double stranded helix are held together by hydrogen bonds between the purine and pyrimidine bases of the respective linear molecules.

Q.48. The degradation of RNA by pancreatic ribonuclease produces:

1. **Nucleoside 2 phosphates**
2. **Nucleoside 3 phosphates**
3. **Nucleoside 5 phosphates**
4. **Nucleotides.**

Ans. 2, 3

The pancreatic enzyme that specifically hydrolyzes ribonucleic acids are ribonucleases. They are capable of cleaving internal phosphodiester bonds to produce either 3-hydroxyl and 5' phosphoryl terminals or 5' hydroxyl and 3' phosphoryl terminals and they are reffered as endonucleases.

Q.49. Restriction of enzymes which have revolutionized the field of genetic engineering have been found only in:

1. **Bacteria**
2. **Humans**
3. **Viruses**
4. **Plants.**

Ans. 1

Restriction enzymes always exists in pairs in a bacterium. They are named after the bacterium from which they were isolated for example- Eco RI for Escherichia coli..

Q.50. Leucine zipper motif is a mediator for:

1. **Membrane attack complexes**
2. **Ligand membranes**
3. **Binding of regulatory proteins to DNA**
4. **Cyclic GMP.**

Ans. **3**

Leucine zipper accounts for many of the specific proteins DNA interactions. Binding must be of high affinity to the specific site and of low affinity to other DNA.

Q.51. Xeroderma pigementosum, a rare skin disease is due to an autosomal recessive trait which causes a deficiency of:

1. **DNA polymerase**
2. **DNA dependent RNA polymerase**
3. **DNA ligase**
4. **A specific DNA endonuclease.**

Ans. **4**

Xeroderma pigmentosum is an autosomal recessive genetic disease. The clinical syndrome includes marked sensitivity to sunlight with subsequent formation of multiple skin cancers and premature death. The inherited defect seems to involve the repair of damaged DNA, particularly thymine dimers.

For treatment endonuclease cut the DNA backbone near the defect, then, after an endonuclease removes a few bases, the defect is filled in by the action of a repair polymerase and the strand is rejoined by a ligase.

Q.52. The attachment site of DNA dependent RNA polymerase to a gene is the:

1. **Operator**
2. **Promoter**
3. **Structural gene**
4. **Regulatory gene.**

Ans. **2**

RNA polymerase associates, with a specific protein factor (the sigma (σ)factor) that helps the core enzyme recognize and binds to the specific DNA sequence of the promoter region to form the preinitiation complex (PIC).

Q.53. Part of mRNA removed during protein synthesis:

1. **Intron**
2. **Codon**
3. **Exon**
4. **Cistron.**

Ans. **1**

The part of mRNA that is transcribed but excised before translation is called intron.

Q.54. Visualization of specific RNA fragment using RNA probe is:

1. **Southern blotting**
2. **Western blotting**
3. **Eastern blotting**
4. **Northen blotting.**

Ans. **4**

Northern blotting is a technique for transferring RNA from an agarose gel to a nitro cellulose filter, on which the RNA can be detected by a suitable probe.

Q.55. To synthesize insulin on a large-scale basis, the most suitable starting material obtained from the beta cells of the pancreas is: **`(AIIMS Nov 2005)**

1. **Genomic DNA**
2. **Total cellular RNA**
3. **cDNA of insulin**
4. **mRNA of insulin.**

Ans. **4**

Insulin is synthesized on large-scale basis from cDNA, but this is not the starting material. The starting material is mRNA. cDNA can be derived from mRNA by following steps-

mRNA (from specific cells of an organism)
↓
mRNA template is annealed to synthetic Oligonucleotide (oligo dT primer)
↓
Reverse transcriptase and dNTP's yield a complementary DNA strand
↓
mRNA - DNA hybrid
↓
mRNA is degraded by alkali
↓
DNA polymarase I and dNTP's yield double stranded DNA
↓
Duplex DNA (cDNA)

This cDNA is inserted into an appropriate cloning vector, which produces large number of cDNA clones. This method is reffered as recombinant DNA technology (RDT).

Q.56. Xeroderma pigmentosum is caused due to a group of closely related abnormalities in: (AIIMS Nov 2005)

1. **Mismatch repair**
2. **Base excision repair**
3. **Nucleotide excision repair**
4. **SOS repair.**

Ans. 3

Xeroderma pigmentosum is a type of skin cancer caused when DNA is constantly being subjected to environmental factors such as radiations or chemicals that cause the alteration or removal of nucleotide bases. If the damage is not repaired a permanent mutation may be introduced that can result in any of a number of deleterious effects including loss of control over the proliferation of the mutated cell, leading to cancer. There are several mechanisms and enzymes, which can repair such type of damage. These repair enzymes are involved in recognizing the lesion, excising the damaged part of the affected DNA strand and using a sister strand as a template to fill the gap left by the excision of the abnormal strand.

Q.57. Apart from occurring in the nucleic acids, pyrimidine is also found in the: (AIIMS Nov 2005)

1. **Theophylline**
2. **Theobromine**
3. **Flavin mononucleotide**
4. **Thiamine.**

Ans. 4

Besides nucleic acids pyrimidine are also found in thiamine. Purine and pyrimidine are the nitrogenous bases found in DNA and RNA. In DNA they are adenine, guanine, cytosine and thiamine and in RNA they are adenine, guanine cytosine and uracil. The structure of thiamine contains a pyrimidine, a thiazole ring and the sulphur.

Q.58. The long and short arms of chromosomes are designated respectively as: (AIPGEE 2006)

1. **p and q arms**
2. **m and q arms**
3. **q and p arms**
4. **I and s arms.**

Ans. 3

The long and short arms of chromosomes are designated respectively as q and p arms. Because the p (petit) is the short arm ad the q (the next letter of the alphabet) is the long arm. When a karyotype is made (actual photograph of chromosome from one cell) the q arm is always put on the bottom and p on the top. A region called centromere separates both the arms. Every cell of the human body has

46 chromosomes occurs in 23 pairs. The last pair of the chromosome is reffered as sex chromosomes labelled as X or Y. In females this pair is designated as (XX) and in males as (XY).

Q.59. Euchromatin is the region of DNA that is relatively: (AIPGEE 2006)

1. **Uncondensed**
2. **Condensed**
3. **Over condensed**
4. **Partially condensed.**

Ans. 2

Euchromatin is the region of the DNA that is relatively condensed.

Transcriptionally inactive chromatin is densely packed during interphase as observed by electron microscopic studies and is reffered to as heterochromatin. Transcriptionally active chromatin stains less densely and is reffered to as euchromatin. Generally euchromatin is replicated earlier then heterochromatin in the mammalian cell cycle.

Q.60. Microsatllite sequence is: (AIPGEE 2006)

1. **Small satellite**
2. **Extra chromosomal DNA**
3. **Short sequence (2-5) repeat DNA**
4. **Looped DNA.**

Ans. 3

Microsatellite repeat sequences consist of one category of repeat sequences exists as both dispersed and grouped tandem arrays. The sequence consists of 2-6 base pairs repeated upto 50 times. These microsatellite sequences most commonly are found as dinucleotide repeats of AC on one strand and TG on the opposite strand, but several other forms occur, including CG, AT and CA. The AC repeat sequences are estimated to occur at 50,000-100,000 locations in the genome. At any locus the number of these repeats may vary on the two chromosomes, thus providing heterozygosity of the number of copies of a particular microsatellite number in an individual.

Q.61. Mitochondrial DNA is: (AIPGEE 2006)

1. **Closed circular.**
2. **Nicked circular.**
3. **Linear.**
4. **Open circular.**

Ans. 1

Human mitochondria contain 2 to 10 copies of a small-closed circular double-stranded DNA molecule that makes up approximately 1% of total cellular DNA. This mt-DNA codes for mt-ribosomal and transfer RNA's and for 13 proteins that plays key roles in the respiratory chain.

An important feature of human mitochondrial mt-DNA is that because the ovum contributes all mitochondria during zygote formation. It is transmitted by the maternal non-Mendelian inheritance.

Thus, in disease resulting from mutations of mt-DNA, an affected mother would in theory pass the disease to all of her children but only her daughters would transmit the trait. However, in some cases, deletions in mt-DNA occur during oogenesis and thus are not inherited from the mother.

Q.62. Which type of RNA is the highest percentage of modified base? (AIPGEE 2006)

1. **mRNA**
2. **tRNA**
3. **rRNA**
4. **snRNA.**

Ans. 2

tRNA has the highest percentage of modified base. It serves as adaptor molecules for the translation of mRNA into protein sequences. The tRNA's contain many modifications of the standard bases A,U,G and C including methylation, reduction, deamination and rearranged glycosidic bonds. Further modification of the tRNA molecule includes nucleotide alkylations and the attachment of the characteristic CpCpAoH terminal at the 3' end of the molecule by the enzyme nucleotidyl transferase.

Q.63. The sigma s subunit of prokaryotic RNA polymerase: (AIPGEE 2006)

1. **Binds the antibiotic rifampicin**
2. **Is inhibited by a amanitin**
3. **Specifically recognizes the promoter site**
4. **Is part of the core enzyme.**

Ans. 3

The sigma s subunit of prokaryotic RNA polymerase specifically recognizes the promoter site. The four subunits of enzyme i.e. 2a, 1b and 1b' are responsible for the 5' ®3' RNA polymerase activity, and are reffered to as the core enzyme. However, this enzyme lacks specificity, that is, it cannot recognize the promoter region on the DNA template. The sigma s subunit enables RNA polymerase to recognize promoter regions of the DNA. The sigma s plus the core enzyme make up the holoenzyme.

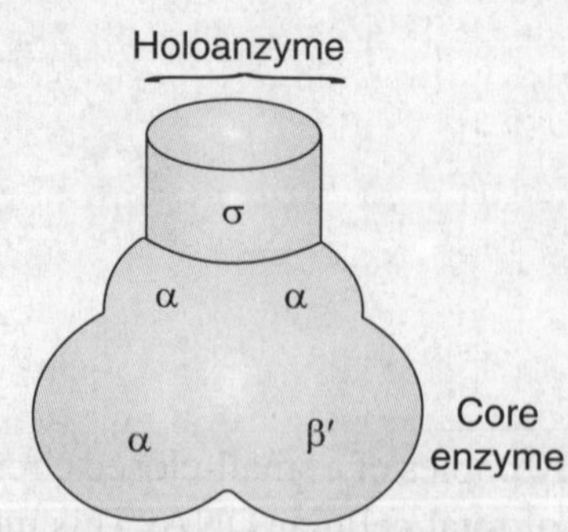

Prokaryotic RNA polymerase

Q.64. Which one of the following is the complementary sequence of 5' TTAAGCTAC 3'? (AIPGEE 2006)

1. **5' GTACGCTTAA 3'**
2. **5' AATTCGCATG 3'**
3. **5' CATGCGAATT 3'**
4. **5' TTAAGCGTAC 3'.**

Ans. 1

As according to Chargaff's rule adenine always pairs with thymine and cytosine always pairs with guanine in equal amount. And complementary sequences of 5'—3' end always proceeds from 3'——5'direction.

Q.65. During replication of DNA, which one of the following enzymes polymerizes the Okazaki fragments? (AIPGEE 2006)

1. **DNA polymerase I**
2. **DNA polymerase II**
3. **DNA polymerase III**
4. **RNA polymerase I.**

Ans. 3

During DNA replication the polymerase III holoenzyme binds to template DNA as part of a multiprotein complex that consists of several polymerase accessory factors. DNA polymerase only synthesizes DNA in the 5' to 3' direction, and only one of the several different types of polymerases is involved at the replication fork. Because the DNA strands are antiparallel, the polymerase functions asymmetrically. On the leading strand (forward) the DNA is synthesized continuously. On the lagging strand (retrograde) the DNA is synthesized in short fragments called Okazaki fragments. To ensure that this happens, the helicase acts on the lagging strand to unwind dsDNA in a 5' to 3' direction. The helicase associates with the primase to afford the latter proper access to the template. This allows the RNA primer to be made and in turn, the polymerase to begin replicating the DNA.

Q.66. All of the cell types contain the enzyme telomerase which protects the length of telomeres at the end of chromosome except: (AIPGEE 2006)

1. **Germinal**
2. **Somatic**
3. **Hemopoietic**
4. **Tumor.**

Ans. 2

The ends of each chromosome contain structures called telomeres. Telomeres consist of short, repeat TG- rich sequences. Human telomeres have a variable number of repeats of the sequence 5'-TTAGGG-3' which can extend for several kilobases. Telomerases, a multisubunit RNA–containing complex related to viral- RNA- dependent DNA polymerases (reverse transcriptase) is the enzyme responsible for telomere synthesis and thus for maintaining the length of the telomere. Since telomere shortening has been associated with both malignant transformation and aging telomerase has become an attractive target for cancer chemotherapy and drug development.

Q.67. Base substitution mutations can have be following molecular consequences except: (AIPGEE 2006)

1. **Changes one codon for an amino acid into another codon for that same amino acid.**
2. **Codon for one amino acid is changed into a codon of another amino acid.**
3. **Reading frame changes downstream to the mutant site.**
4. **Codon for one amino acid is changed into a translation termination codon.**

Ans. 3

Base substitution mutation	Frame shift mutation
Involves changes to a single base (point mutations) and substitution of the base with another base. May be seen as- Transitions: pyrimidine changed to pyrimidine. Transversion: purine to pyrimidine or vice versa.	Involves change to a single base but no substitution. May be seen as: Deletion and insertion.
The resulting mRNA will show a change only at the point complementary to a base change at the corresponding locus.	The resulting mRNA shows a major alteration downstream to the mutant site, because the translating machinery does not recognize that a base was missing.
Effects	**Effects**
1. Silent mutation:- change in base in mRNA on third nucleotide of a codon usually causes no detectable effect because degeneracy of the code. (change one codon for an amino acid into another codon for the same amino acid).	1. Garbled translation of the mRNA all the way distal to the single nucleotide deletion.
2. Missense effect: A different amino acid is incorporated at the corresponding site in the protein molecule. (codon for one amino acid is changed into codon for another amino acid).	2. Premature termination may occur if reading of the message results in appearance of a nonsense codon.
3. Nonsense effect:-A nonsense codon can appear that would then result in premature termination of peptide chain and only a fragment of the intended protein will be produced (codon for one amino acid is changed into translation termination codon).	

Q.68. The following methods can be used to detect the point mutation in the beta globin gene that causes sickle cell anemia, except: (AIPGEE 2006)

1. Polymerase chain reaction with allele specific Oligonucleotide hybridization

2. Southern blot analysis

3. DNA sequencing

4. Northern blot analysis.

Ans. 4

Polymerase chain reaction, DNA sequencing and southern blot testing are rapid methods for DNA analysis, and can all be used to detect the point mutation in the globin gene. Whereas the northern blot is the technique to analyze RNA rather than DNA.

Q.69. A nucleic acid was analyzed and found to contain 32% adenine, 18% guanine, 17% cytosine and 33% thymine. The nucleic acid must be: (AIIMS May 2006)

1. Single stranded RNA

2. Single stranded DNA

3. Double stranded RNA

4. Double stranded DNA.

Ans. 4

According to Chargaff's rule in double stranded DNA, amount of adenine is always equal to thymine and amount of cytosine is always equal to guanine.

Q.70. The following are the generalized diagram of the typical eukaryotic gene:

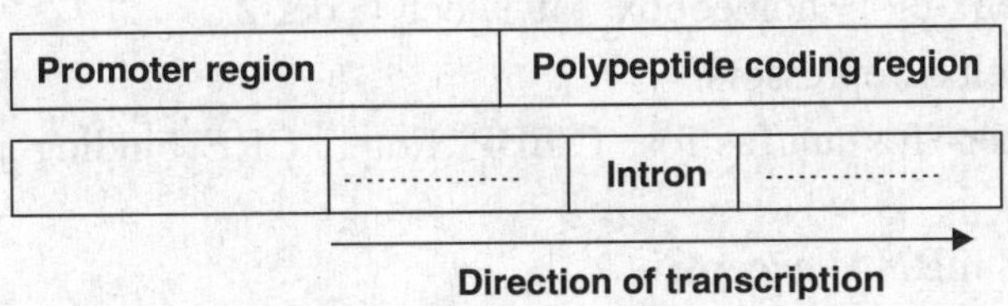

What is the most likely effect of a 2 base pair insertion in the middle of the intron? (AIIMS May 2006)

1. Normal transcription, altered translation

2. Defective termination of transcription, normal translation

3. Normal transcription, defective mRNA splicing

4. Normal transcription, normal translation.

Ans. 4

mRNA is initially transcribed as a long, exact copy of the DNA strand, but posttranslational processing results in retention of the essential information needed for translation to protein. The genome contains introns, which interrupt the coding sequences, the exons. The intron material does not contain information for translation, so it must be removed for translation. This occurs during the

RNA processing step, which is regulated by conserved sequences that identify the end and start of the exons, allowing the coding portions to be spliced together. Because the signals that lead to removal are not stringent, it is possible for exons to be occasionally skipped and for spliced variants and splice mutations to occur. This gives a great degree of flexibility for the final gene product and allows tissue- specific products.

Q.71. Steroids binds to a regulatory protein, on DNA through: (AIIMS Nov 2006)

1. **Zinc finger motif**
2. **Leucine zipper motif**
3. **Helix turn helix**
4. **Helix loop helix.**

Ans. 1

Steroids such as estrogen, due to their hydrophobic nature, diffuse across the cell membrane. Within the cell, estrogen binds to the highly specific soluble receptor proteins, called as nuclear hormone receptors. They have two highly conserved domains, i.e. a DNA binding domains and a ligand-binding domain. DNA binding domain lies towards the centre of the molecule and provides these receptors with sequence specific DNA binding sites. Zinc ions stabilizes the structure of these domains, hence such domains are often reffered to as zinc finger domains.

The second highly conserved region of the nuclear receptor protein is reffered to as the ligand-binding site. On binding of the ligand (signal molecule), ligand- receptor complex modifies the expression of the specific genes, by binding to control elements in the DNA.

DNA binding domains are of four types:

1. Helix turn helix-eg- ,homeobox, pit-1, oct 1, oct-2.
2. Helix loop helix- repressors.
3. Leucine zipper- fos-jun/fos-fos, C/EBP, Fra-1, CRE binding protein, c-myc, n-myc, l-myc.

Q.72. All are true of mRNA except: (AIPGEE 2007)

1. **Capping helps in attachment of mRNA to 40S ribosome**
2. **In eukaryotes is regulated by GTP to GDP transformation**
3. **The first amino acid is methionine**
4. **Synthesized from DNA 3'———5'.**

Ans. 3

mRNA is synthesized from a DNA template by the enzyme RNA polymerase in 3'——5' direction. The translation (conversion of mRNA to protein) is completed under three steps:-

1. Initiation
2. Elongation
3. Termination

In eukaryotes the initiation factors- namely IF_1 and IF_3 – first bind with free 30 S subunit. This is followed by the attachment of mRNA with 30S subunit in presence of GTP. The 50S ribosomes associates with 30S to form 70 S initiation complex and the initiation factors are released. During this process GTP is con verted to GDP with the release of pyrophosphate. The 5' end of the mRNA is capped with 7-Methyl guanosine by an unusual 5'——5' triphosphate linkage. This cap is required for translation, besides stabilizing the structure of mRNA.

Q.73. Northern blot is used for the analysis of: **(AIPGEE 2007)**

1. **mRNA expression**
2. **DNA**
3. **Protein**
4. **None of the above.**

Ans. 1

The northern and western blot transfer techniques are used to size and quantitate specific RNA and protein molecules, respectively. Another hybridization technique, the south western blot, examines protein- DNA interactions. Proteins are separated by electrophoresis, renatured, and analyzed for an interaction by hybridization with a specific labeled DNA probe.

Q.74. Study of gene expression is called: **(AIPGEE 2007)**

1. **Proteinomics**
2. **Proteonomics**
3. **Genomics**
4. **Geneomics.**

Ans. 3

Genomics is the study of an organisms entire genome. A major branch of genomics is still concerned with sequencing the genomes of various organisms. Although the knowledge of full genomes have created the possibility for the field of functional genomics, mainly concerned with patterns of gene expression during various conditions.

Q.75. Lac operon ________? **(AIPGEE 2007)**

1. **Negative regulator**
2. **Positive regulator**
3. **Repression**
4. **Derepression.**

Ans. 1

The lac operon consists of a regulatory gene, operator gene and three structural genes. Besides these genes, there is a promoter site, next to the operator gene, where the enzyme RNA polymerase binds. Lac repressor is a tetrameric regulatory protein, which specifically binds to the operator gene. This prevents the binding of the enzyme RNA polymerase to the promoter site. Thereby blocking the transcription of the structural genes. The repressor molecule acts as negative regulator of gene expression.

Q.76. All of the following acts on the nucleus via transcription factors:(AIPGEE 2007)

1. **Insulin**
2. **Vitamin D**
3. **Retinoids**
4. **All of the above.**

Ans. 1

NOTES

12

Starvation

1. Fuel reserve present in a well nourished man is: 1600 kcal in glycogen, 24,000 kcal in mobilizable protein and 1,35,000 kcal in triacylglycerol.
2. The major amino acid transported from muscle to liver during starvation: Alanine
3. The metabolic fuel during prolonged fasting is: Ketone bodies.
4. During starvation, the compounds that degrade sequentially to meet energy needs are: Liver glycogen, triacylglycerol of adipose tissue, muscle proteins.
5. During starvation, fuels available are utilized in order as: Ketone bodies, free fatty acid, glucose.
6. The pathways stimulated during starvation are: Gluconeogenesis, glycogenolysis, lipolysis, β-oxidation, ketogenesis, muscle protein breakdown.
7. The pathways down regulated during starvation are: Glycogenesis, HMP shunt, lipogenesis, cholesterol biosynthesis.
8. Fatty liver is seen during starvation because of: Less α - glycero-P, VLDL formation and elimination leading to accumulation of fat.
9. The need for drinking water is reduced due to: Increase in metabolic water & relative expansion of ECF by reduced glomerular filtration.

SOLVED QUESTIONS

Q.1. Energy source used by brain in later days of starvation is: (AIPGME 1994)

1. Glucose

2. Ketone bodies

3. Glycogen

4. Fatty acids.

Ans. 2

During first 2 to 3 days of starvation energy is obtained from glycogenolysis. Stored liver glycogen is utilized for energy production. Gluconeogenesis from glucogenic amino acids also occurs. After this first stage, in the second stage, stored fat is mobilised. Fat depots of the adipose tissue is broken into free fatty acids which are oxidised for energy production. This second stage lasts for two weeks. Acetyl coA produced by fatty acid oxidation is utilised for ketone body production These ketone bodies are then utilized for energy purpose.

Q.2. If starvation exceeds 7 days , the major nutritional supply of the brain comes from: (AIPGME 1995)

1. **Fatty acids**
2. **Ketone bodies**
3. **Protein breakdown**
4. **Carbohydrate breakdown.**

Ans. 2

If starvation exceed 7 days as the stored glycogen is already utilized during first 2-3 days of starvation, the body has to start utilizing stored fat. This fat is broken down to fatty acids which are then oxidized for energy production. Acetyl coA is chanelled to ketone body production.

Q.3. In a patient with starvation for 72 hours which of the following would be seen: (AIIMS MAY 2002)

1. **Increased glycogenolysis**
2. **Increased ketosis due to break down of fats**
3. **Degradation of proteins**
4. **Increased gluconeogenesis.**

Ans. 2

Explanation same as Q.1. Once the body fat is totally exhausted degradation of tissue protein starts.

13

Xenobiotics

1. Xenobiotics: Foreign molecules which enter the body.
2. Types of Detoxification: (Phase I - oxidation, reduction, hydroxylation, (Phase II - conjugation).
3. The enzyme system involved in the hydroxylation reactions is: Cytochrome P450.
4. Site of xenobiotics metabolism: Liver, endoplasnic reticulum.
5. Various conjugating agents are: Glucuronic acid, S-adenosyl methionine, acetyl coA, sulfuric acid, amino acids (Glycine, L-Cysteine), glutamine, thiosulfate, glutathione.
6. Example of a substance that can exists in procarcinogen form and is activated by cytochrome P 450 enzyme is: Polycyclic aromatic hydrocarbon.
7. Aspirin is hydrolysed to: Acetic acid + Salicylic acid.
8. The drug Isoniazid, used in treatment of TB is detoxicated by: Acetylation.
9. Example of conjugation with glucuronic acid is: Conjugation of bilirubin to form bilirubin diglucuronide.
10. Benzoic acid is detoxified by: Conjugation with glycine: It forms hippuric acid.
11. Aromatic compounds are detoxified by conjugation with L- cysteine in presence of acetic acid to form: Mercapturic acid.
12. Selenium poisoning can be cured by administering: P-Bromobenzene.
13. A detoxicant used for certain war poisons is: Dithiopropanol (2, 3-Mercaptopropanol).
14. Major lipid found in cytochrome P 450 is: Phosphatidylcholine.

SOLVED QUESTIONS

Q.1. In Cytochromes P-450, P stands for: **(AIPGME 1999)**

1. Structural protein

2. Polymer

3. Substrate protein
4. Pigment.

Ans. 4

Cytochrome P-450 is considered the most versatile biocatalyst. Hydroxylation reactions of detoxification are catalysed by cytochrome P-450 or monooxygenases. They are the major monooxygenases in the endoplasmic reticulum. They are so named because the enzyme was discovered when it was noted that preparations of microsomes that had been chemically reduced and then exposed to carbon monoxide exhibited a distant peak at 450 nm.

Q.2. The main enzyme responsible for activation of xenobiotics is: (AIPGME 2003)

1. Cytochromes P-450
2. Glutathione S-transferase
3. NADPH Cytochromes P-450 reductase
4. Glucuronyl transferase.

Ans. 1

Cytochromes P-450 is mostly utilized for hydroxylation of xenobiotics. But induction of cytochromes P-450 system may even produce unwanted effects in some persons. Xenobiotics may be converted to harmful compounds by the cytochromes P-450 dependent oxygenase. Example is polycyclic aromatic hydrocarbon exists in procarcinogen form and is activated by cytochromes P- 450 system.

Q.3. Detoxification of drugs is controlled by:

1. Cytochrome
2. Cytochrome P^{450}
3. Cytochrome C
4. Cytochrome A.

Ans. 2

Cytochrome P^{450} are called so because the enzyme was discovered when it was noted that preparations of microsomes that had been chemically reduced and then exposed to carbon monoxide exhibited a distinct peak at 450 nm. It is important as approximately 50% of the drugs human ingest are metabolized by isoforms of cytochrome P^{450}, these enzymes also act on various carcinogens and pollutants.

14 Nutrition

1. The energy content of food materials is measured in: Calories.
2. The energy yielding nutrients are: Carbohydrates, fats, proteins.
3. Calorific value of nutrients (The quantity of energy provided by nutrients is):
   Carbohydrates - 4 Kcal/g.
   Fats - 9 Kcal/g
   Proteins - 4 Kcal/g
   Alcohol - 7 Kcal/g.
4. Respiratory quotient is: The ratio of volume of CO_2 produced to the O_2 consumed.
5. R.Q of different nutrients is:
   Carbohydrates - 1.
   Fats - 0.7
   Proteins - 0.8.
6. For a mixed diet R.Q is between: 0.7 and 1.
7. R. Q is lowest in: Active ketolysis [when rate of utilisation of fat increases in relation to carbohydrate, RQ falls].
8. While calculating the energy requirements of an individual the factors to be considered are:
   (1) Basal metabolic rate
   (2) Specific dynamic action of food
   (3) Physical activity
   (4) Thermogenesis when atmospheric temperature is low.
9. Basal metabolic rate is proportional to: Lean body weight and surface.
10. Specific dynamic action refers to: Increased heat production following the intake of food (thermogenic effect of food).
11. Specific dynamic action of important nutrients is: Protein has highest S.D.A. about 30% while fat has 4% and carbohydrates has 6%.

12. Dietary fibers include: Cellulose, hemicellulose, lignin, pectins, mucilage.
13. High protein quality refers to: High percentage of essential amino acids.
14. The high quality proteins that are used as reference: Egg and milk proteins standards are.
15. Increased fiber in the diet reduces incidence of: Diverticulosis, CA colon, D.M. atherosclerosis.
16. Kwashiorker results from: Deficiency of protein.
17. Marasmus results from: Deficiency of both dietary energy and proteins.
18. Minimum recommended daily carbohydrate intake to prevent ketosis is: 50-100 g.

SOLVED QUESTIONS

Q.1. Dietary fibre contains: **(AIPGME 1996)**

1. **Collagen**
2. **Pectin**
3. **Proteoglycans**
4. **Starch.**

Ans: **2**

The unavailable or indigestible carbohydrate in the diet is called dietary fibre.These include cellulose, hemicellulose, lignin, pectins, mucilage. Dietary fibre is necessary to maintain the normal motility of gastrointestinal tract.

Q.2. Following constitute dietary fibres except: **(AIPGME 1999)**

1. **Pectin**
2. **Cellulose**
3. **Hemicellulose**
4. **Riboflavin.**

Ans: **4**

Explanation same as Q.1

Q.3. Nitrogen to caloric ratio in total parenteral nutrition is: **(AIIMS June 2000)**

1. **1 gm of N_2: 150 non protein calories**
2. **1 gm of N_2: 100 non protein calories**
3. **1.25 gm of N_2: 100 non protein calories**
4. **1.25 gm of N_2: 150 non protein calories.**

Ans: **1**

A healthy adult at rest requires 1500-2000 non protein kilo calories. Mostly energy is provided by carbohydrates and fats. Each gm of carbohydrate and fat provides about 4.1 k cal and 9.1 k cal of energy respectively. So about 150 k cal: 1gm relation i.e 2000 k cal:13 gN is present.

Q.4. Cereal and Pulse are complementary in protein diet because:

1. **Cereal contain 10% protein and pulse contain 20% protein**
2. **Cereal lacks lysine and pulse lacks methionine**
3. **Cereal protein has non-essential amino acids**
4. **Pulso protein has essential amino acids.**

Ans: 2

Pulses are deficient in methionine, while cereals lack in lysine. A Vegetable protein lacking a particular essential amino acid, if supplemented by another vegetable protein possessing that amino acid and taken simultaneously, the biological value of each of these two low- quality proteins is enhanced.

NOTES

NOTES

15 Muscle Tissue and Connective Tissue

1. The major muscle proteins are: Actin, myosin, troponin, tropomyosin.
2. Most abundant muscle protein: Myosin.
3. The major protein of the thin filaments, actin; can polymerise into a fibrous form called: F-actin.
4. The muscle contraction is modulated by troponin and tropomyosin through: Ca^{2+}.
5. Calcium binding proteins in striated muscle are: Troponin -C, Calsequestrin.
6. A meshwork of actin filaments and spectrin is attached to the plasma membrane by: Ankyrin.
7. A Calmodulin associated protein which increases spectrin binding to actin is: Adducin.
8. Tau proteins (brain microtubules) and caldesmon (smooth muscle) are collectively referred to as: Flip-Flop switch proteins.
9. Calcium binding protein in smooth muscle: Calmodulin.
10. Major energy reserve in muscle: Creatine phosphate.
11. White muscle do not contain: Myoglobin.
12. Muscle contraction is effected by: The sliding of actin over myosin.
13. Components of connective tissue are: Proteins and glycosaminoglycans.
14. Protein in connective tissue are: Collagen, elastin, fibronectin, fibrillin and laminin.
15. The major structural protein found in connective tissue: Collagen.
16. Most abundant amino acid in collagen: Glycine.
17. Most abundant collagen in body: Type-I collagen.
18. Collagen is synthesized by fibroblasts intracellularly on: Membrane bound ribosomes.
19. Collagen on boiling looses viscosity and gets converted to an altered protein called: Gelatin.
20. Elastin is synthesized from: Tropoelastin.
21. Accumulation of elastin is associated with: Scleroderma.
22. High levels of laminin have been reported in patients suffering from: Alzheimer's disease.

General feature of inherited diseases that affect collagen

Disease	Clinical Feature	Biochemical Causes
Osteogenesis imperfecta	Abnormal fragility of bones	Various abnormalities in genes coding for procollagen α – i(1)
Ehlers Danlos Syndrome	Hyper mobile joints skin abnormalities	Abnormality in gene for procollagen α-1(III) deficiency of lysyl hydroxylase deficiency of procollagen N- proteinase
Marfan's Syndrome	Skeletal, ocular and cardio-vascular abnormalities	Mutation in gene for fibrillin
Menke's Syndrome	Kinky hair, growth retardation	Lysyl oxidase deficiency due to abnormal copper metabolism

SOLVED QUESTIONS

Q.1. In collagen synthesis, hydroxylation of proline to hydroxyproline requires all except:

1. **Pyridoxal phosphate**
2. **Vitamin C**
3. **Oxygen**
4. **Dioxygenase.**

Ans: 1

In collagen synthesis, hydroxylation of proline to hydroxyproline residue is a post translational modification taking place intracellularly. The enzyme is prolyl hydroxylase is a di-oxygenase which uses molecular oxygen. The enzyme requires a reducing agent like ascobric acid. Pyridoxal phosphate is a coenzyme of transamination reactions

Q.2. All of the following are required for required for hydroxylation of proline in collagen synthesis except:

1. **O_2**
2. **Vitamin C**
3. **Dioxygenase**
4. **Pyridoxal phosphate.**

Ans: 4

Explanation same as Q.1

Q.3. The collagen triple helix structure is not found in:

1. **Cytoplasm**
2. **Golgi apparatus**

3. **Lumen of endopasmic reticulum**
4. **Intracellular vesicles.**

Ans: **1**

Newly synthesized collagen undergoes post translational modification before becoming part of a mature extracellular collagen fiber. Collagen is synthesized on ribosomes and further modifications occurs in golgi apparatus like hydroxylation of proline and lysine residues. Intrachain and interchain disulfide bond formation assists in the formation of collagen triple helix. This triple helix is then secreted from the cell by way of the golgi apparatus in intracellular vesicles.

Q.4. Keratin of skin and nail differ because of:

1. **Disulphide bond**
2. **Covalent bond**
3. **Van der waals bond**
4. **Hydrogen bond**

Ans: **1**

Keratins are fibrous proteins. They are rich in cysteine which are responsible for covalent disulphide bonds between adjacent polypeptide chains.These bonds are responsible for rigidity so the number of disulphide bonds affect the rigidity. Keratins are the major component of skin, hair and nail. The difference between keratin of skin and nail is in the rigidity of the structure i.e. the number of disulphide bonds between the polypeptide chain differs.

Q.5. Collagen is rich in:

1. **Glutamate and glycine**
2. **Alanine and glycine**
3. **Proline and glycine**
4. **Glutamate and proline.**

Ans: **3**

The R groups of each polypeptide strand of the triple helix pack so closely that in order to fit, one must be glycine. Thus every third amino acid residue in collagen is a glycine residue. Collagen is also rich in proline and hydroxyproline, yielding a repetitive Gly-x-y- pattern in which y generally is proline or hydroxyproline.

NOTES

16 Liver, Thyroid and Renal Function Tests

1. The basic tests in any suspected liver disease: Estimations of total and conjugated bilirubin.
2. When there is rise in conjugated bilirubin the reaction is: Direct positive.
3. An increase in both conjugated and unconjugated bilirubin is seen in: Hepatocellular jaundice.
4. Complete absence of faecal urobilinogen is strongly suggestive of: Malignant obstruction.
5. Appearance of jaundice on the 2nd and 3rd day after birth is: Physiologic jaundice.
6. Clay colored pale stools are seen in: Post hepatic obstructive jaundice.
7. Certain drugs such as chlorpromazine causes: Cholestatic jaundice.
8. The monosaccharide used to assess metabolic capacity of liver is: Galactose.
9. In advanced parenchymal liver disease or cirrhosis of liver: Hypoalbuminemia and associated hypergammaglobulinemia causing reversal of A : G ratio.
10. Galactose tolerance test with slow fall in blood is suggestive of: Parenchymal liver disease.
11. For differential diagnosis of jaundice, enzyme used is: Alkaline phosphatase.
12. Characteristic of hepato biliary disease is: 5'– Nucleotidase.
13. Marker enzyme in chronic alcoholism is: Gamma glutamyl transpeptidase.
14. The basis of laboratory diagnosis of thyroid diseases is: Measurement of T_4 and T_3 levels in blood.
15. The precursor amino acid of thyroid hormones is: Tyrosine.
16. In primary hypothyroidism TSH level is elevated and T_3 and T_4 are low.
17. Cholesterol level in hyperthyroidism is: Decreased.
18. Euthyroid goiter can result from: Iodine deficiency.
19. The substances which prevent iodine uptake or utilization by thyroid gland are: Goitrogens.
20. The compounds having goitrogenic effect are: Thiooxazolidone, thiocyanate, iso–thiocyanate, polyphenolic glycosides.
21. Amount of urine excreted in 24 hrs is; 1.5 L.
22. The glomerular filtration rate is about: 120 – 125 ml/min or 170 – 175 l/day.

23. Classification of renal function tests is based upon: GFR, renal plasma flow and tubular function.
24. Clearance of a substance is defined as: The volume of plasma completety cleared of that substance in 1 min.
25. Stepwise increase in uric acid, urea and creatinine reflect: Kidney dysfunction.
26. Inulin clearance is a measure of: GFR.
27. Daily excretion of urea is: 25 – 30 Gm.
28. Nonprotein – nitrogenous constituents of urine are: Urea, uric acid, ammonia, creatinine, hippuric acid.
29. Concentration and dilution tests are employed to assess: Tubular function.
30. Compounds whose excretion in urine are dependent on blood level are known as: Threshold substances.
31. Large quantities of albumin are lost in urine in: Nephrosis.
32. Microalbuminuria is seen as a complication of: Diabetes mellitus and hypertension.
33. Phenol sulphonphthalein (PSP) is used to test: Tubular secretory capacity.
34. Fanconi's syndrome is: Non-specific amino aciduria with excessive excretion of substances as carbohydrate and phosphate.

17

Miscellaneous

Q.1. Function of metabolism includes all except: (AIPGME 1994)

1. Extraction of nutrients from food

2. Breakdown of substrate

3. Equilibrium of biochemical with intracellular components

4. Using building blocks for synthesis.

Ans. 1

The fate of dietary components after digestion and absorption constitutes metabolism – The metabolic pathways taken by individual molecules, their interrelationships and the mechanisms that regulate the flow of metabolites through the pathways.

Metabolic pathways fall into three categories

(I) Anabolic pathways – involved in the synthesis of compounds

(II) Catabolic pathways -involved in the breakdown of larger molecules

(III) Amphibolic pathways – acting as links between the anabolic and catabolic pathways.

Q.2. Which of the following is luminous? (AIPGME 1994)

1. Porphyrin

2. Zymogen

3. Chromatin

4. Albumin.

Ans. 1

The various porphyrins are all coloured. Each exhibits the characteristic absorption spectrum in both the visible and the ultraviolet regions of the spectrum. When porphyrins dissolved in strong mineral acids are illuminated by u.v light, they emit a strong red fluorescence. Zymogens are the inactive precursor proteins. It is easy to rule out the other options chromatin and albumin.

Q.3. A protein estimation test is confused with: (AIPGME 1996)

1. **Phosphates**
2. **Nitrates**
3. **Sulphates**
4. **Bile salts.**

Ans. **1**

The proteinuria is commonly assessed by the heat and acetic acid test proteins are coagulated on heating and precipitated at the isoelectric point when acetic acid is added. Calcium phosphates and magnesium phosphates are also precipitated on boiling but they are soluble in acidic medium.

Q.4. Strongest bond amongst the following is:

1. **Hydrophobic**
2. **Electrostatic**
3. **Hydrogen bond**
4. **Vander waal's forces.**

Ans. **2**

Electrostatic bonds are the attractive forces between two opposite charges or repulsion between two like charges. Solubility of such compound in polar solvents is much higher because a large amount of energy (energy of hydration) is released when ions tightly bind water molecules. Hydrogen bonds are formed by sharing of a hydrogen atom between two electron donors. The strength of a hydrogen bond in water is much weaker than a covalent bond between oxygen and hydrogen.

Hydrophobic interactions are the interactions between non-polar hydrophobic side chains by eliminating water molecule van der waal's forces are very weak forces of attraction between polar and non- polar molecules.

Q.5. True statement regarding covalent bonds is: (AIPGME 1996)

1. **Electrons have same spin**
2. **Electrons have opposite spin**
3. **They are weak bonds**
4. **None of the above.**

Ans. **2**

The covalent bond is the strongest force that holds molecules together. Sharing of electrons occur between the atoms and the electrons always have a opposite spin in the orbitals.

Q.6. All of the following statements are correct about metabolism in brain except: (AIPGME 1998)

1. **Fatty acids are utilized in starvation**
2. **60% of total energy is utilised during resting stage**
3. **Ketone bodies are used in starvation**
4. **Has no stored energy.**

Ans. 1

There is no stored fuel in the brain. Glucose the preferred fuel for the brain, should be in continuous supply. Glucose can freely enter the brain cells. The total consumption of glucose by brain is about 120 g/day (420 k cal). Thus about 60%of the total carboyhydrate intake by the body is metabolized by the brain. The brain is unable to utilize fatty acids as a source of fuel since the fatty acids complexed to albumin are unable to traverse the blood brain barrier However, brain can effectively utilize acetoacetate. This is a survival technique in diabetic and starvation ketosis.

Q.7. Strongest bond out of the following is: (AIPGME 1998)

1. **Electrostatic**
2. **Hydrogen**
3. **Hydrophobic**
4. **Van der waal's.**

Ans. 1

Explanation same as Q.4

Q.8. A destitute woman is admitted to the hospital with altered sensorium and dehydration; urine analysis slows mild proterinuria and no sugar; what other test would be desirable:

1. **Fouchet**
2. **Rothera**
3. **Hays**
4. **Benedict's.**

Ans. 2

Q.9. The following separation technique depends on the molecular size of the protein: (AIPGME 2003)

1. **Chromatography on a carboxymethyl (CM) cellulose column**
2. **Isoelectric focusing**
3. **Gel filtration chromatography**
4. **Chromatogrphy on a diethylaminoethyl (DEAE) cellulose medium.**

Ans. 3

In gel filtration chromatography, hydrophilic cross linked gels like acrylamide, agarose and dextran are used for separation of molecules based on their size. The gel particles are porous in nature. Gel particles of specific pore size are selected for isolation of that specific sized protein Chromatography on CM-cellulose or on a DEAE – cellulose medium is based on electrophoretic attraction between charged biological molecules to oppositely charged groups on the ion exchange resins. Iso electric focussing is a electrophoretic technique and is based on pH gradient

Q.10. The conversion of an optically pure isomer (Enantiomer) into a mixture of equal amounts of both dextro and levo forms is called as: (AIPGME 2003)

1. **Polymerization**
2. **Stereo isomerization**
3. **Racemization**
4. **Fractionation.**

Ans. **3**

A mixture of equal amounts of both dextro and levo form is called recemic mixture. As equal amount of both the forms are present their optical rotations cancel each other hence their mixture (racemic mixture) is optically inactive. The process of conversion of enantiomer into a mixture of equal amounts of both dextro and levo forms is called racemization.

Q.11. The substance present in gall bladder stones or the kidney stones can be best identified by the following techniques: (AIPGME 2003)

1. **Fluorescence spectroscopy**
2. **Electron microscopy**
3. **Nuclear magnetic resonance**
4. **X-ray diffraction.**

Ans. **4**

X-ray diffraction – refers to the diffraction of X- rays by a crystal . The wavelengths of x-rays are comparable in size to the distances between atoms in most crystals and repeated pattern of crystal lattice acts as a diffraction grating for X- rays. The application of crystallographic techniques such as electron microscopy, energy dispersive elemental analysis and x-ray diffraction have established the role of different microcrystals including monosodium urate, calcium pyrophosphate dihydrate calcium hydroxyapatite in inducing arthritis or periarthritis.

Q.12. Proteins targeted for destruction in eukaryotes are covalently linked to: (AIPGME 2004)

1. **Clathrin**
2. **Pepsin**
3. **Laminin**
4. **Ubiquitin.**

Ans. **4**

Degradation of abnormal and other short lived proteins occurs in the cytosol and requires ATP and ubiquitin. Ubiquitin is a small (8.5 k Da) protein that targets many intracellular proteins for degradation. Several molecules of ubiquitin are attached by non α-peptide bonds formed between the carboxyl terminal of ubiquitin and the ε - amino group of lysyl residues in the target protein .

Q.13. Which of the following is not a rate limiting enzyme: (AIIMS DEC 1998)

1. **HMG coA reductase**
2. **Phosphofructokinase**

3. Acetyl CoA carboxylase
4. Malonate dehydrogenase.

Ans. **4**

HMG co A reductase is the rate limiting enzyme of cholesterol biosynthesis. Acetyl co A carboxylase is the rate limiting enzyme of fatty acid synthesis. Phosphofructokinase is the key regulatory enzyme of glycolytic pathway.

Q.14. Molecular size is assessed by: (AIIMS DEC 1998)

1. Sedimentation
2. Absorption mass spectroscopy
3. Liophilization
4. Salting out.

Ans. **1**

Molecular weight (size) can be determined in an ultracentrifuge. Larger molecules can be sedimented at high centrifugal forces whereas small molecules cannot . Rate of sedimentation depends on the size , shape and density of solute particles. Spectroscopy technique is used for structural analysis of glycoproteins. Lyophilisation is the process by which water is evaporated at very low temperature in vaccum. It is a process of protein preservation.

Salting out is a method of protein precipitation. In this method the shell of hydration present around the protein molecule is removed by adding a salt solution.

Q.15. In human body, the action of surfactant is done by: (AIIMS MAY 2001)

1. Sugar and salt
2. Soap and water
3. Lipid and protein
4. Base and lipid.

Ans. **3**

Surfactant molecules are amphipathic i.e they possess both polar group and nonpolar chain. Amphipathic nature is required for its action. Such a combination is present in phospholipids and proteins. Thus surfactant is made up of – Dipalimitoyl phosphatidyl choline, phosphatidyl glycerol, other phospholipids, neutral lipids, proteins and carbohydrate.

Q.16. In chromatography mass movements of the substances is due to: (AIIMS MAY 2001)

1. Diffusion
2. Electrophoresis
3. Paper chromatography
4. Osmosis.

Ans. **1**

Q.17. In which type of chromatography, the proteins are bound to another substance: (AIIMS MAY 2001)

1. **Hydrophobic chromatography**
2. **Affinity chromatography**
3. **Paper chromatography**
4. **Gel chromatography.**

Ans. 2

Affinity chromatography is based on the high affinity of specific proteins for specific chemical groups. Thus coenzymes can be used to purify enzymes.

Q.18. The presence of 2 extra pairs of electrons on the oxygen in water molecule results in: (AIIMS MAY 2002)

1. **Makes water a non-polar solvent**
2. **Forms covalent bonds in the ice**
3. **Electro negative charge on water molecule**
4. **Electro positive charge on water molecule.**

Ans. 3

The presence of extra pair of electron (e^-) impart a electronegative charge, not positive charge. Water molecule has tetrahedron shape. Along with that it possess 2 extra pairs of electrons so water becomes a electrical dipole, the oxygen atom bearing a negative charge (2^-) and each hydrogen having a positive charge (1^+).

Q.19. The following separation technique depends on the molecular size of protein: (AIIMS NOV 2002)

1. **Chromatography on a carboxy methyl (CM) cellulose column**
2. **Isoelectric focussing**
3. **Gel filtration chromatography**
4. **Chromatography on a diethyl amino ethyl (DEAE) cellulose column.**

Ans. 3

Hydrophilic cross linked gels like acrylamide, agarose and dextran are used for separation of molecules based on their size. The range of separation is based on pore size. These pores will allow small molecules enter into the gel. But larger molecules could not enter into the pores of the gel.

18

Practice Questions

Q.1. Which of the following fatty acids is found exclusively in breast milk ?

1. Linoleic
2. Linolenic
3. Palmitic
4. Dacosahexaenoic acid.

Q.2. True about increased HDL / LDL ratio is:

1. It increases circulating TG
2. It decreases TG in blood
3. It increases esterification of circulating cholesterol
4. It leads to down regulation of ApoB receptor.

Q.3. How many ATP's are formed in case of stearic acid by β oxidation ?

1. 7
2. 129
3. 56
4. 146.

Q.4. Triglyceride synthesis is increased by:

1. Growth hormone
2. Insulin
3. Cortisol
4. Glucagon.

Q.5. Erythrocyte membrane has:

1. Lactosyl ceramide
2. Beta sulfogalactocerebroside
3. Glucocerebroside
4. Galactocerebroside.

Q.6. Triacylglycerols:

1. Would be expected to be good emulsifying agents
2. Yield about the same amount of ATP on complete oxidation as would an equivalent weight of glycogen
3. Are stored as hydrated molecules
4. In the average individual, represent sufficient energy to sustain life for several weeks

Q.7. Which subcellular fraction of mammalian hepatocytes contain the enzymes necessary for elongation of long chain fatty acid ?

1. Plasma membrane
2. Nucleus
3. Endoplasmic reticulum
4. Organelle- free cytosol.

Q.8. The cyclization of squalene in mammals results in the direct formation of which of the following sterols:

1. Cholesterol
2. Desmosterol
3. Lanosterol
4. Sitosterol.

Q.9. Rats fed a fat free diet from birth would be deficient in:

1. Sphingolipids
2. Phospholipids
3. Triacylglycerols
4. Prostaglandins.

Q.10. Hypercholesterolemia is commonly associated with:

1. Thyrotoxicosis
2. Obstructive jaundice
3. Infective hepatitis
4. Glycogen storage diseases.

Q.11. A two stage cholesterol method involving the Lieberman Burchardt reaction is susceptible to interference from:

1. Proteins
2. Other sterols
3. Lipaemia
4. Bilirubin.

Q.12. All of the following inhibit platelet aggregation except:

1. Thromboxane A2
2. Prostacyclin

3. Aspirin
4. Benoxaprofen.

Q.13. Phosphatides occur in:

1. Myelin sheath
2. Stabilizes chylomicrons
3. In erythrocyte membrane
4. All above.

Q.14. Sphingosine is backbone of all of the following except:

1. Cerebroside
2. Ceramide
3. Sphingomyelin
4. Lecithin

Q.15. Which of the following is more effective in inhibiting HMG CoA reductase ?

1. VLDL
2. LDL
3. HDL
4. IDL.

Q.16. 12 years old boy is brought to the hospital with a case of easy bruising, bleeding associated with mass in the abdomen. Bone marrow examination reveals pancytopenia and lots of foam cells. The likely disorder in this patient is:

1. Gauchers' disease
2. Metachromatic leukodystrophy
3. Krabbe's disease
4. Fabry's disease.

Q.17. Proteins and lipopolysaccarides are carried in blood in:

1. LDL
2. HDL
3. VLDL
4. Chylomicron.

Q.18. The following is the shorthand representative of archidonic acid:

1. 20 : 4; 5, 8, 11, 14
2. 18 : 3 ; 9, 12, 15
3. 18 : 2; 9, 12
4. 16 :1; 1.

Q.19. The normal concentration of lipids in the liver is around:

1. 5%
2. 10%

3. 15%
4. 20%.

Q.20. The ratio of esterified cholesterol to free cholesterol in circulation is around:

1. 1:1
2. 2:1
3. 3:1
4. 1:3.

Q.21. The rate limiting enzyme in bile salt synthesis is:

1. HMG-CoA reductase
2. HMG-CoA synthetase
3. 7- alpha- hydroxylase
4. Decarboxylase.

Q.22. Primary bile acids:

1. Are any bile acids that are found in the intestinal tract
2. Are any bile acids reabsorbed from the intestinal tract
3. Are synthesized in the intestinal tract by bacteria
4. Are synthesized in hepatocytes directly from cholesterol
5. Are converted to secondary bile acid by conjugation with glycine or taurine.

Q.23. Truly essential fatty acid is:

1. Oleic acid
2. Linoleic acid
3. Linolenic acid
4. Arachidonic acid.

Q.24. Levostatin acts by:

1. HMG CoA reductase inhibition
2. Inhibiting mevalonate kinase
3. Inhibiting cholesterol absorption
4. Metabolizing cholesterol.

Q.25. The ketone which contributes maximally to diabetic ketoacidosis is:

1. Acetone
2. Acetoacetic acid
3. Pyruvate
4. Beta- hydroxybutyrate.

Q.26. Which of the following has a ketogenic effect on liver ?

1. Glucagon
2. Insulin

3. Androgen
4. Growth hormone.

Q.27. Following are true of protein clathrin except:

1. Coating of pits and vesicles
2. Octapeptide with quaternary structure
3. Involved in cell structure maintenance
4. Endocytosis protein.

Q.28. Thromboxane A2 is mostly produced by:

1. Platelets
2. Endothelium
3. Damaged tissues
4. WBC.

Q.29. Stored triacylglycerol in adipose tissue is released by:

1. Lysosomal lipase
2. Lipoprotein lipase
3. LCAT
4. Hormone sensitive lipase.

Q.30. Fatty acids with even carbons cannot be converted to carbohydrates in the body, as one of the following reactions is not possible:

1. Glucose-6-phosphate to glucose-1-phosphate
2. Fructose-1,6-bisphosphate to fructose -6- phosphate
3. Acetyl CoA to pyruvate
4. Fatty acid to Acetyl CoA.

Q.31. Apo B 48 and Apo B 100 are expressed as two different apoprotein because of difference in:

1. RNA editing
2. RNA splicing
3. Chromosomal loci
4. Apo-B gene.

Q.32. The number of mevalonate molecules required for synthesis of one molecule of cholesterol are:

1. 2
2. 4
3. 5
4. 6.

Q.33. Cholesterol present in LDL:

1. Represents primarily cholesterol that is being removed from peripheral cells
2. Binds to a receptor and diffuses across the cell membrane

3. On accumulation in the cell inhibits replenishment of LDL receptors
4. When enters a cell , suppresses activity of acyl Co A: Cholesterol acyltransferase.

Q.34. The net yield of high energy bonds from the complete oxidation of acetoacetate in the brain is:

1. 11
2. 12
3. 23
4. 24

Q.35. The release of arachidonate from membrane glycerophospholipids is inhibited by which one of the following compounds:

1. Aspirin
2. Linoleic acid
3. A specific protein induced by glucocorticoids
4. 2-acyl lysophosphatidylcholine

Q.36. Detergent action of bile salts is due to:

1. Amphipathic property
2. Acts as zwitterions
3. Hydropathic property
4. All of the above.

Q.37. What happens to the lipid bilayer on adding unsaturated fatty acid to it ?

1. Fluidity decreases
2. Fluidity increases
3. Non predictable effect on fluidity
4. No effect.

Q.38. Following is rich in linoleic acid:

1. Ground nut oil
2. Linseed oil
3. Soyabean oil
4. Sun flower oil.

Q.39. Which of the following undergoes auto oxidation ?

1. FFA
2. PUFA
3. Chylomicrons
4. Cholesterol.

Q.40. In fatty acid synthesis, which of the following is required:

1. Niacin
2. Pantothenic acid

3. Biotin
4. All of the above.

Q.41. $C_{17}H_{27}COOH$ is formula of:

1. Linoleic acid
2. Linolenic acid
3. Arachidonic acid
4. Clupanodonic acid.

Q.42. The half life of free fatty acid in plasma is:

1. 5-10 minutes
2. 1-2 minutes
3. 30 minutes
4. 60 minutes.

Q.43. Which of the following mainly transports fatty acids from adipose tissue to other tissue for metabolism ?

1. Carnitine
2. Chylomicrons
3. Plasma albumin
4. High density lipoprotein.

Q.44. Fatty acid synthase:

1. Yields an unsaturated fatty acid by skipping a reductive step
2. Produces hydroxyl fatty acids in nerve tissue
3. Can stop with the release of a fatty alcohol instead of an acid
4. Can produce a branched chain fatty acid if methylmalonyl Co A is used as a substrate.

Q.45. Phospholipases A_1 and A_2:

1. Are responsible for the initial insertion of fatty acids in Sn-1 and Sn-2 positions during synthesis
2. Are responsible for base exchange in the interconversion of phosphatidylethanolamine and phosphatidylserine
3. Hydrolyse phosphatidic acid to a diaglyceride
4. Remove a fatty acid in a Sn-1 or Sn-2 position so it can be replaced by another in phospholipids synthesis.

Q.46. Which of the following is not a major reaction occurring in the hepatocytes ?

1. Bile pigment synthesis
2. Esterification of cholesterol
3. Transamination
4. Glycogenolysis.

Q.47. Experimental atherosclerosis may be produced in monkeys by:

1. Pyridoxine deficiency
2. Riboflavin deficiency
3. Vit. E deficiency
4. Feeding riboflavin and arachidonic acid.

Q.48. Hydroperoxyeicosa tetraenoic acid (HPETE'S):

1. Are derived from arachidonic acid by a peroxidase reaction
2. Are intermediates in the formation of leukotrienes
3. Are relatively stable compounds
4. Are inactivated forms of leukotrienes.

Q.49. Roles of various phospholipids include all of the following except:

1. Cell – cell recognition
2. A surfactant functions in lung.
3. Activation of certain membrane enzymes
4. Mediator of hypersensitivity and acute inflammatory reactions.

Q.50. Which of the following type of hyperlipoproteinemia is seen associated with pancreatic insufficiency:

1. Type-I
2. Type-II
3. Type-IV
4. Type-V.

Q.51. Which of the following enzymes catalyze reactions in the biosynthesis of both catecholamines and indoleamines (serotonin) ?

1. Dopamine β-hydroxylase
2. Phenyl ethanolamine N-methyl transferase
3. Aromatic amino acid Decarboxylase
4. Tryptophan hydroxylase.

Q.52. Which of the statements about protein structure is true ?

1. The extended β-configuration is not found in globular proteins
2. The stability of alpha- helix is mainly due to hydrophobic interactions
3. Globular proteins tend to fold into configurations that keep hydrophobic side chains in the interior of the molecule
4. The primary structure of a peptide does not influence the formation of native 3 dimensional configurations.

Q.53. Ammonium ion is released by:

1. Arginase
2. Glutamate dehydrogenase

3. Glutaminase
4. All above.

Q.54. The human plasma proteins are a mixture of:

1. Glycoproteins
2. Simple proteins
3. Conjugated proteins
4. All above.

Q.55. Peptidases require the presence of following for their action:

1. Mo
2. Mn
3. Co
4. Cu.

Q.56. Following amino acids participate in transamination reaction except:

1. Alanine
2. Lysine
3. Aspartate
4. Glutamate.

Q.57. Creatine is formed metabolically from:

1. Tryptophan
2. Arginine
3. Phenylalanine
4. Histidine.

Q.58. The term secondary structure of proteins refers to as:

1. Alpha helix and beta pleated sheets
2. Overall confirmations
3. Subunit interactions
4. Relationship of two polypeptide chains.

Q.59. Amino acid not stable in alpha helix is:

1. Proline
2. Alanine
3. Glutamine
4. Tryptophan.

Q.60. Semi essential amino acids are:

1. Arginine and Histidine
2. Cysteine and glycine
3. Phenylalanine and tyrosine
4. Threonine and arginine.

Q.61. Homogentisate oxidase is an:

1. Oxidase
2. Mono oxygenase
3. Dioxygenase
4. Anaerobic dehydrogenase.

Q.62. RNA which determines amino acid sequences:

1. m RNA
2. t RNA
3. r RNA
4. All above.

Q.63. The amino acid that can proteinate and deproteinate at neutral pH is:

1. Glycine
2. Proline
3. Serine
4. Histidine.

Q.64. Taurine is mainly formed from amino acid:

1. Glycine
2. Lysine
3. Cysteine
4. Histidine.

Q.65. All of the following are proteins except:

1. Heparin
2. Insulin
3. Mucin
4. Pepsin.

Q.66. Chains A and B of insulin contains __amino acids respectively:

1. 30, 21
2. 21, 31
3. 31, 20
4. 20, 31.

Q.67. Histidine is synthesized from:

1. Glutamate
2. Aspartate
3. Ribose-5-phosphate
4. Serine.

Q.68. Which of the following amino acids gives yellow color with ninhydrin in paper chromatography ?

1. Alanine
2. Proline
3. Tryptophan
4. Tyrosine.

Q.69. Which amino acid undergoes transamination to form α-keto isocaproic acid ?

1. Valine
2. Threonine
3. Lysine
4. Leucine

Q.70. Which of the following is a derived protein ?

1. Protamines
2. Peptones
3. Prolamines
4. Lactalbumin.

Q.71. Choline, a most important lipotropic factor is formed with the help of following except:

1. Methionine
2. Serine
3. Glycine
4. Histidine.

Q.72. One of the following amino acids contribute hydrophobic properties to the protein:

1. Serine
2. Leucine
3. Histidine
4. tyrosine.

Q.73. Tamm Horsfal protein is secreted by:

1. Proximal tubules of ascending limb of Henle
2. Distal tubules of ascending limb of Henle
3. Distal tubules of descending limb of Henle
4. Proximal tubules of descending limb of Henle.

Q.74. Negative nitrogen balance is produced in humans by elimination from the diet of all of the following amino acids except:

1. Leucine
2. Methionine
3. Lysine
4. Serine

Q.75. The most abundant protein in the human body is:

1. Myosin
2. Albumin
3. Hemoglobin
4. Keratin.

Q.76. Which of the following amino acids has an isoionic point of approximately physiological Ph ?

1. Glycine
2. Arginine
3. Lysine
4. Histidine.

Q.77. Noncovalent interactions in a protein may be disrupted by:

1. Dinitrophenol
2. Mercaptoethanol
3. Cyanogenbromide
4. Guanidine hydrochloride.

Q.78. The amino acid with two asymmetric carbon atoms:

1. Valine
2. Serine
3. Tryptophan
4. Isoleucine.

Q.79. All of the following procedure are useful in determination of amino acid sequence except:

1. Edman degradation
2. Racemization
3. Chymotropic digestion
4. Reaction with 2,4-DNFB.

Q.80. Carnitine is synthesized from:

1. Lysine and Methionine
2. Leucine and isoleucin
3. Malonyl CoA and glycerol phosphate
4. Glycine and arginine.

Q.81. Serum albumin:

1. Has the highest molecular weight, on the average, of serum proteins
2. Makes the largest contribution to the osmotic pressure of serum
3. Plays a major role in the transport of triacylglycerol and Cholesterol esters
4. Binds to bilirubin and calcium.

Q.82. Vibrational spectrum of proteins is due to structure:

1. Primary
2. Secondary
3. Tertiary
4. Quaternary.

Q.83. Bence Jones proteins are:

1. Light chains
2. Heavy chains
3. Cryoglobulins
4. C- reactive proteins.

Q.84. Glycoproteins is:

1. HCG
2. Glucagon
3. Insulin
4. All of the above.

Q.85. For phosphorylation , amino acids is:

1. Serine
2. Cysteine
3. Glycine
4. Alanine.

Q.86. Amino acid mediating flexibility of proteins is:

1. Glycine
2. Tryptophan
3. Phenylalanine
4. Histidine.

Q.87. The most abundant glycoprotein present in basement membrane is:

1. Laminin
2. Fibronectin
3. Collagen type 4
4. Heparan sulphate.

Q.88. Aminotransferases:

1. Usually require α- ketoglutarate or glutamine as one of the reacting pair
2. Catalyze reactions that result in a net use or production of amino acids
3. Require pyridoxal phosphate as an essential cofactor for the reaction
4. Are not able to catalyze transamination reactions with essential amino acids

Q.89. Glutathione does all of the following except:

1. Scavenge peroxides and free radicals

2. Form sulfur, conjugates for detoxication of compounds
3. Convert hemoglobin to methaemoglobin
4. Act as a cofactor for some enzymes.

Q.90. Carbamoyl phosphate synthetase-I:

1. Is controlled primarily by feed back inhibition
2. Is unresponsive to changes in arginine
3. Requires N-acetyl glutamate as an allosteric effectors
4. Requires ATP as an allosteric effectors.

Q.91. Sullivan reaction is done for detection of:

1. Arginine
2. Tyrosine
3. Tryptophan
4. Cysteine.

Q.92. Constituent of gelatin is:

1. Hydroxylysine
2. β- Alanine
3. Ornithine
4. Phenylalanine.

Q.93. True statement about the peptide bond:

1. C-C bond
2. Cis – hydrogen and O_2 group
3. It is planar
4. Rotational freedom.

Q.94. Hydrogen bonds in the secondary and tertiary structure of proteins are directly attacked by:

1. Salts
2. Detergents
3. Alkali
4. All above.

Q.95. Ergothionine is derived from amino acids:

1. Histidine
2. Glycine
3. Isoleucine
4. Tyrosine.

Q.96. __gm of N2 is lost per day in a normal adult:

1. 1-3
2. 3-5

3. 5-7
4. 7-9.

Q.97. Which absorb light in proteins:

1. Peptide bonds
2. Prosthetic group
3. Aromatic amino acids
4. Nodular groups.

Q.98. Defect in folding of the protein result in which of the following clinical disease:

1. Kuru
2. Migraine
3. Hypothyroidism
4. Myopia.

Q.99. Increased risk of myocardial infarction is associated with which amino acid:

1. Methionine
2. Homocysteine
3. Ornithine
4. Valine

Q.100. Which of these amino acids migrate slowest to the anode at the physiological Ph ?

1. Aspartic acid
2. Glycine
3. Lysine
4. Valine.

Q.101. Carbohydrate not having even a single asymmetric carbon atom:

1. Dihydroxyacetone
2. Erythrose
3. Ribose
4. Glucose.

Q.102. Fucose is a:

1. Triose
2. Hexose
3. Methyl pentose
4. Glycoside.

Q.103. Iodine solution produces no colour with:

1. Starch
2. Dextrin
3. Glycogen
4. Cellulose.

Q.104. Predominant mucopolysaccharide of cartilage is:

1. Hyaluronic acid
2. Collagen
3. Elastin
4. Chondroitin sulphate.

Q.105. Best test for blood glucose estimation:

1. Glucose oxidase method
2. Folin-Wu method
3. Orthotoluidine method
4. Hexokinase method.

Q.106. Which one of the following human tissue contains greatest amount of the body glycogen ?

1. Liver
2. Kidney
3. Skeletal muscle
4. Adipose tissue.

Q.107. A deoxy-sugar characteristic of blood group polysaccharides is:

1. L-Rhamnose
2. L-Fucose
3. 2-deoxy-D-ribose
4. 6-deoxy-L-mannose.

Q.108. The key regulatory enzyme of the Pentose Phosphate Pathway is positively regulated by:

1. NADH
2. ADP
3. GTP
4. $NADP^+$
5. FADH.

Q.109. Among following ___ is not a glycosaminoglycan:

1. Collagen
2. Hyaluronic acid
3. Chondroitin sulphate
5. Keratan sulphate.

Q.110. Insulin increases the activities of all of the following enzymes, Except:

1. Glucokinase
2. Pyruvate carboxylase
3. Glycogen synthase
4. Acetyl-CoA carboxylase.

Q.111. Skeletal muscle is deficient in:

1. Glucose-6-phosphatase
2. Hexokinase
3. Isomerase
4. Phosphofructokinase.

Q.112. Insulin receptors are:

1. Tyrosine kinase receptors
2. Phosphodiesterase
3. Calcium-calmodulin
4. Lipoprotein lipase
5. All.

Q.113. Insulin helps in all Except:

1. Glycogen synthesis
2. Gluconeogenesis
3. Lipogenesis
4. Glycolysis.

Q.114. Inhibition of glycolysis by O_2 is called:

1. Crabtree effect
2. Hill reaction
3. Pasteur effect
4. Gluconeogenesis.

Q.115. Under anaerobic conditions of glycolysis one molecule of glucose yields___ molecules of ATP:

1. 1
2. 6
3. 2
4. 30.

Q.116. Most important ion in glycolysis is:

1. Calcium
2. Manganese
3. Copper
4. Magnesium.

Q.117. Which does not occur in glycolysis ?

1. Isomerisation
2. Hydration
3. Phosphoryl transfer
4. All above.

Q.118. Substrate level phosphorylation is seen in the conversion of:

1. Acetoacetate to a-ketoglutarate
2. Succinyl CoA to Succinate
3. Fumarate to Malate
4. Succinate to Fumarate.

Q.119. Acetyl CoA is least used in the synthesis of which of the following in a well fed state:

1. Citrate
2. Acetoacetate
3. Oxalosuccinate
4. Palmityl CoA.

Q.120. Formation of citrate from oxaloacetate and acetyl CoA is:

1. Reduction
2. Oxidation
3. Condensation
4. Hydrolysis.

Q.121. Malate shuttle is important in:

1. Glycogenolysis
2. HMP
3. Glycolysis
4. Gluconeogenesis.

Q.122. Rate limiting step in Kreb's cycle is mediated by:

1. Citrate synthase
2. Isocitrate dehydrogenase
3. Succinate dehydrogenase
4. Malate dehydrogenase.

Q.123. The amphibolic pathway among the following is:

1. TCA
2. Glycogenesis
3. Lipolysis
4. Glycolytic.

Q.124. The rate of absorption of sugars by small intestine is highest for:

1. Disaccharides
2. Polysaccharides
3. Hexoses
4. Pentoses.

Q.125. The only sugar absorbed by small intestine against a concentration gradient is:

1. Glucose
2. Galactose
3. Mannose
4. Xylose.

Q.126. The main products of HMP shunt are all Except:

1. 6 $NADPH_2$
2. 2 Fructose-6-phosphate
3. 1 Glyceraldehyde-3-phosphate
4. 1 CO_2.

Q.127. NADPH is required for:

1. HMP shunt
2. Glycolysis
3. Fatty acid synthesis
4. Glycogenolysis.

Q.128. The end product of citric acid cycle used in detoxification of ammonia in brain is:

1. Oxaloacetate
2. α-ketoglutarate
3. Succinate
4. Citrate.

Q.129. Glucose can be synthesized from all of the following Except:

1. Acetoacetate
2. Lactic acid
3. Glycerol
4. Amino acid.

Q.130. Gluconeogenesis occurs in liver and:

1. Kidney
2. Muscle
3. Heart
4. Lactating mammary gland.

Q.131. Epinephrine can bring about the glycogenolysis in:

1. Liver
2. Muscle
3. None
4. Liver and Muscle.

Q.132. __ is common to both glycogenesis and glycogenolysis:

1. Glucose-1-phosphate

2. Hydration of pyrophosphate
3. Both use the same enzyme for branching and debranching
4. All above.

Q.133. __ form of glycogen synthase is dependant on the presence of Glucose-6-phosphate for full activity:

1. D
2. L
3. Both
4. None.

Q.134. In glycogen, the branches are formed by a1,6 links at approximately every ___ glucose unit:

1. 10
2. 12
3. 14
4. 16.

Q.135. Von Gierke's disease is due to deficiency of enzyme ___

1. Glucose – 6-phosphatase
2. Glucose – 1-phosphatase
3. Phosphorylase
4. Branching enzyme.

Q.136. Ratio of insulin/glucagons causes:

1. ↓ Ratio of cAMP / 5 AMP
2. ↓ Levels of lipoprotein lipase
3. ↓ Amino acid synthesis
4. all above.

Q.137. UDP-Glucuronic acid is required for the biosynthesis of:

1. Glyogen
2. Chondroitin Sulphate
3. Lactose
4. Starch.

Q.138. Galactosemia commonly is due to deficiency of:

1. Galactose – 1 – phosphate uridyl transferase
2. Galactose – 1 – phosphatase
3. Glucose – 1 – phosphatase
4. Glucose – 6 – phosphatase.

Q.139. A patient suffering from galactosemia are placed on a galactose free diet. Galactose, however, is required by the body to form brain cerebrosides. How is galactose formed in patients on a galatose free diet ?

1. Epimerisation of uridine diphosphate (UDP)glucose
2. Reaction of a 5- and a 4 – carbon sugar catalysed by transketolase
3. Reaction of a 7- and a 3 – carbon sugar catalysed by transaldolase
4. Reaction of two 3 – carbon sugars catalysed by aldolase
5. Oxiadation of sorbitol.

Q.140. An otherwise asymptomatic patient exhibits hemolytic anemia after treatment with antimalarial drug primaquine. What metabolic process is not functioning normally in this patient ?

1. Pentose phosphate pathway
2. Uronic acid pathway
3. Metabolism of amino sugars
4. Galatose metabolism
5. Fructose metabolism.

Q.141. Repeating disaccharide unit in cellulose is:

1. Dextrin
2. Sucrose
3. Cellobiose
4. Maltose.

Q.142. Hereditary fructose intolerance is caused due to deficiency of:

1. Phosphofructokinase
2. Fructokinase
3. Phosphofructoaldolase
4. Triose phosphate isomerase.

Q.143. Transketolase actlvity is affected in:

1. Biotin deficiency
2. Pyridoxine deficiency
3. Thiamine deficiency
4. Manganese deficiency.

Q.144. Certain amino sugars may be components of:

1. DNA
2. Glycogen
3. ABO blood group antigens
4. Vitamin C

Q.145. Isomers formed as a result of interchange of –OH and -H ions on carbon atoms 2, 3, 4 of glucose are known as:

1. Optical isomers
2. Anomers
3. Epimers
4. Aldose-ketose isomers.

Q.146. Which type of glycogenesis is transmitted by X linked genes ?

1. Type I
2. Type II
3. Type III
4. Phosphorylase B kinase.

Q.147. In the synthesis of which compound nucleotide sugars are not involved ?

1. Ganglioside
2. Glycoprotein
3. Proteoglycan
4. Sphingomyelin.

Q.148. Deficiencies of all the following enzymes result in enlarged liver and hypoglycemia Except:

1. Amylo (1, 4 $\rightarrow$ 1, 6) transglycosylase
2. Phosphorylase
3. Phosphorylase kinase
4. Amylo 1 $\rightarrow$ 6 glucosidase.

Q.149. Mitochondrial membrane has transporter for:

1 NADH
2 ATP- ADP transport
3 Galactose
4. cAMP.

Q.150. Deficiency of vitamin___ produces methylmalonic aciduria:

1. Vitamin A
2. Vitamin C
3. Vitamin B_{12}
4. Riboflavin.

Q.151. The two polynucleotide chains of DNA double helix:

1. Are connected by disulphide bonds
2. Are held together by phosphate diester bonds
3. Cannot be separated
4. Differ in chemical composition.

Q.152. mRNA is a complementary copy of:

1. tRNA
2. rRNA
3. Ribosomal RNA
4. Single strand of DNA.

Q.153. Conversion of UMP to TMP requires:

1. ATP
2. Tetrahydrofolic Acid
3. FMN
4. Pyridoxal phosphate.

Q.154. Complete acid hydrolysis of nucleic acids will not yield:

1. Ribose
2. Guanine
3. Phosphate
4. Adenosine

Q.155. Ribosomal RNA:

1. Accounts for greater part of all the RNA present in the cell
2. Complimentary to mitochondrial DNA
3. Contains amino acid activating enzyme
4. Identical to tRNA.

Q.156. Xeroderma pigmentosum, a rare skin disease is due to an autosomal recessive trait, which causes a deficiency of:

1. DNA polymerase
2. DNA dependent RNA polymerase
3. DNA ligase
4. A specific DNA endonuclease.

Q.157. The smallest unit of DNA capable of regulating the synthesis of a polypeptide is the:

1. Operon
2. Cistron
3. Recon
4. Muton.

Q.158. The percentage of a bacterial chromosome usually involved in transformation is:

1. 1 percent
2. 10 percent
3. 25 percent
4. 50-100 percent.

Q.159. Actinomycin D interferes with enzyme induction by combining with:

1. tRNA
2. rRNA
3. DNA
4. Negative feedback inhibition system.

Q.160. What is the average number of high energy bonds required for the synthesis of 1 peptide bond ?

1. 5
2. 4
3. 2
4. 3

Q.161. Because of the properties of the genetic code:

1. Mutations corresponding to the first base of a codon rarely lead to a substitution of one amino acid for another
2. There are only 20 codons that correspond to each of the encoded amino acids
3. There is a single termination codon
4. In many instances mutations involving the third base of a codon lead to no change in protein structure.

Q.162. Which of the following is a substrate for ribonucleotide reductase in the production of deoxyribonucleotides in humans ?

1. ATP
2. AMP
3. TDP
4. GTP.

Q.163. Jacob and Monod postulated that enzyme inducers exert their effect by interacting with:

1. Operator gene
2. Repressor protein
3. Structural gene
4. Regulatory metabolite

Q.164. Replacement of purine for purine and pyrimidine for pyramidine is called:

1. Transversion
2. Transition
3. Translocation
4. Transcription.

Q.165. Independent DNA replication occurs in all except:

1. Bacteria
2. Mitochondria

3. Nuclei
4. Viruses.

Q.166. If the percentage of adenine in a double stranded DNA molecule is 20%, the percentage of guanine is:

1. 10%
2. 20%
3. 30%
4. 60%.

Q.167. Which of the following is incorporated directly into the polypeptide chain during the translation of mRNA ?

1. Asparagine
2. Homoserine
3. 4 – hydroxyproline
4. Phosphoserine

Q.168. All of the following enzymes are involved in the excision repair of DNA except:

1. DNA Ligase
2. DNA glycocyclase
3. Exonuclease
4. DNA β – polymerase.

Q.169. Gene transmitted but not translated is:

1. Histone
2. Keratin
3. t RNA
4. Glycosyl.

Q.170. Both strands of DNA serve as templates concurrently in:

1. Replication
2. Excision repair
3. Mismatch repair
4. Transcription couple repair.

Q.171. ___contains both a 7 methylguanosine triphosphate cap and a polyadenylate segment:

1. m RNA
2. hn RNA
3. r RNA
4. Sn RNA.

Q.172. The sigma (σ) subunit of prokaryotic RNA polymerase:

1. Is part of the core enzyme
2. Binds the antibiotic rifampicin

3. Is inhibited by α-amanitin
4. Specifically recognizes promoter sites.

Q.173. Degeneracy of the genetic code denotes the existence of:

1. Multiple codons for a single amino acid
2. Codons consisting of only two bases
3. Base triplets that do not code for any amino acid
4. Different protein synthesis systems in which a given triplets codes for different amino acids.

Q.174. Requirements for eukaryotic protein synthesis include all of the following except:

1. mRNA
2. Ribosomes
3. 20 different amino acids in the form of aminoacyl-t RNA's
4. F met - tRNA.

Q.175. Diphtheria toxin:

1. Acts catalytically
2. Releases incomplete polypeptide chains from the ribosomes
3. Activates translocase
4. Prevents release factor from recognizing termination signals.

Q.176. Development of recombinant DNA methodologies is based on discovery of:

1. The polymerase chain reaction (PCR)
2. Restriction endonucleases
3. Plasmids
4. Complementary DNA (cDNA).

Q.177. Full expression of the lac operon requires:

1. Lactose and cAMP
2. Allolactose and cAMP
3. Lactose alone
4. Allolactose alone.

Q.178. All of the following describe an operon except:

1. Control mechanism for eukaryotic genes
2. Includes structural genes
3. Expected to code for polycistronic mRNA
4. Contains control sequences such as an operator.

Q.179. The code word of which protein is also an initiation code for proteins:

1. Leucine
2. Isoleucine

3. Methionine
4. Lysine.

Q.180. Which cell organelle contains DNA ?

1. Mitochondrion
2. Golgi body
3. Endoplasmic reticulum
4. Centriole.

Q.181. Shine- Dalgarno sequence in bacterial mRNA is near:

1. AUG codon
2. UAA codon
3. UAG codon
4. UGA codon.

Q.182. A segment of an eukaryotic gene that is not represented in the mature mRNA, is known as:

1. Intron
2. Exon
3. Plasmid
4. TATA box.

Q.183. RNA polymerase II is involved in the transcription of:

1. hn RNA
2. tRNA
3. 45S rRNA
4. 5S rRNA.

Q.184. Which of the following helps to relieve the supercoils and torques in the unwinding DNA duplex ?

1. DNA topoisomerases
2. DNA helicases
3. Rep protein
4. DNA polymerase III.

Q.185. Northern blot test is used for:

1. DNA analysis
2. RNA analysis
3. Analysis of protein
4. Enzyme analysis.

Q.186. The carbon atom in deoxyribose that contains one oxygen less than ribose is:

1. 3

2. 2
3. 4
4. 1.

Q.187. An increased melting temperature (Tm) for duplex DNA results from a high content of:

1. Adenine + Guanine
2. Cytosine + Thymine
3. Adenine + Thymine
4. Cytosine + Guanine.

Q.188. In a mutation, if Valine is replaced by which of the following, would not result in any change in the function of protein:

1. Proline
2. Leucine
3. Glycine
4. Aspartic acid.

Q.189. Which of the following antibiotics can not be used for treatment because it is accepted as an analog of aminoacyl tRNA by both bacterial and human cells:

1. Erythromycin
2. Tetracycline
3. Streptomycin
4. Puromycin.

Q.190. The correct sequence of cell cycle is:

1. G_0-G_1-S-G_2-M
2. G_0-G_1-G_2-S-M
3. G_0-M-G_2-S-G_1
4. G_0-G_1-S-M-G_2.

Q.191. The mother has sickle cell disease, father is normal, chances of children having sickle cell disease and sickle cell trait respectively are:

1. 0% and 100%
2. 25% and 25%
3. 50% and 50%
4. 10% and 50%.

Q.192. What is the possible cause for gout in a patient who has a glucose -6- phosphatase deficiency ?

1. Increased synthesis of pentoses
2. Increased accumulation of sorbitol

3. Increased synthesis of glycerol
4. Decreased function of Krebs's cycle

Q.193. Committed step in de novo synthesis of purine nucleotides is formation of:

1. Ribose- 5- phosphate
2. 5´-phosphoribosyl-1-pyrophosphate
3. 5´-phosphoribosylamine
4. 5-phosphoribosylglycinamide.

Q.194. All of the following can be used to detect mutation, except:

1. Single strand conformational polymorphism
2. Ligase chain reaction
3. Polymerase chain reaction
4. cDNA sequencing.

Q.195. Null mutation is:

1. Mutation occurring in noncoding region
2. Mutation that eliminates gene function
3. Mutation that codes for a change in progeny without any chromosomal damage
4. None of the above.

Q.196. Leucine zipper motif is a mediator for:

1. Membrane attack complexes
2. Receptor ligand protein
3. Binding of regulatory protein to DNA
4. B-cells epitopes.

Q.197. The synthesis of peptide chain begins at the:

1. N-terminal
2. C-terminal
3. Sugar group
4. Phosphate end.

Q.198. Which one of the following has catalytic activity ?

1. Nucleotides
2. Phospholipids
3. Glycogen
4. RNA.

Q.199. Which of the following is an antiapoptotic gene ?

1. C-myc
2. p53
3. Bcl-2
4. Bax.

Q.200. At the physiological pH the DNA molecules are:

1. Positively charged
2. Negatively charged
3. Neutral
4. Amphipathic.

Q.201. The common feature of enzyme cascade systems is:

1. Amplification
2. Feedback inhibition
3. Allosteric inhibition
4. counter regulation.

Q.202. Specific poison for succinate dehydrogenase is:

1. Arsenic
2. Cyanide
3. Malonate
4. Fluoride.

Q.203. Which of the following enzymes do not need cofactor ?

1. Oxidoreductase
2. Isomerase
3. Aldolase
4. Lyases.

Q.204. Abzyme is:

1. Alloenzyme
2. Isoenzyme
3. Artificially synthesized antibody with catalytic action
4. Prosthetic group.

Q.205. 5`-Nucleotidase activity is increased in:

1. Bone disease
2. Prostate cancer
3. Chronic renal failure
4. Cholestatic disorders.

Q.206. Enzymes catalyze reactions by:

1. Increasing entropy of a system
2. Altering reaction equilibria
3. Lowering total energy levels of reactants
4. Decreasing free energy of activation.

Q.207. If curve X in the graph below represents no inhibition for the reaction of some enzyme with its substrate, which of the other curves would represent competitive inhibition of the same reaction ?

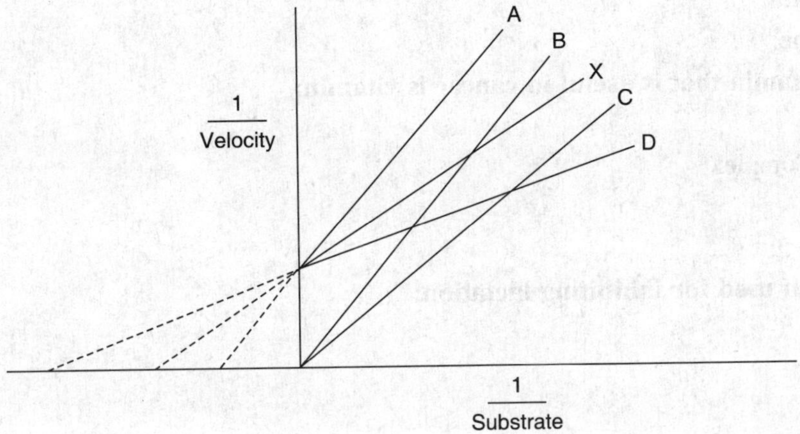

1. A
2. B
3. C
4. D.

Q.208. Enzymes E_a, E_b and E_c are under allowsteric control of S_2, P_1 and P_2 respectively. If E_c is defective what would occur;

1. Accumulation of S_1
2. Accumulation of P_1
3. Accumulation of S_2
4. Decrease of S_2

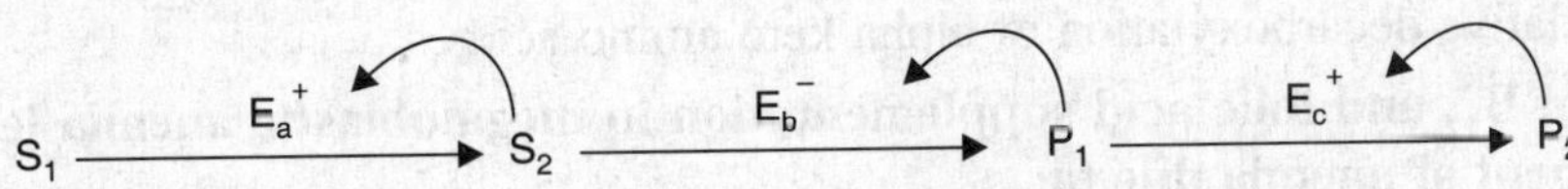

Q.209. Which vitamin is found as a constituent of warburg yellow ?

1. B_1
2. B_2
3. Niacin
4. Pantothenic acid.

Q.210. Growth of bacteria requiring P-aminobenzoic acid is inhibited by:

1. Penicillin
2. Citrovorum factor
3. Tetrahydrofolic acid
4. Sulphonamides.

Q.211. Feeding an avidin may result in a deficiency of:

1. Vitamine A
2. Vitamine B_{12}
3. Biotin
4. None.

Q.212. The vitamin that is useful in cancer is vitamin:

1. A
2. B-Complex
3. C
4. E.

Q.213. Vitamin used for inhibiting lactation:

1. B_1
2. B_2
3. B_6
4. B_{12}.

Q.214. Both vitamin K and C are involved in:

1. The synthesis of clotting factors
2. Post translational modifications
3. Antioxidant mechanisms
4. Microsomal hydroxylation reactions.

Q.215. Thiamine is not used in which of the following rections:

1. Lactate to pyryvate
2. Alphaketoglutarate to succinyl CoA
3. Glucose to pentose
4. Oxidative decarboxylation of alpha keto amino acids.

Q.216. Vitamin B_{12} and folic acid supplementation in megaloblastic anemia leads to the improvement of anemia due to:

1. Increased DNA synthesis in bone marrow
2. Increased Hemoglobin production
3. Erythroid hyperplasia
4. Increased iron absorption.

Q.217. Which of the following must be modified to serve as a cofactor for enzymes ?

1. Copper
2. Biotin
3. Zinc
4. Pantothenic acid.

Q.218. Iron is mainly absorbed in:

1. Stomach
2. Duodenum
3. Lower jejunum
4. Ileum.

Q.219. Substantial quantity of which of the following inorganic ion is required for ribosomal function:

1. Cu^{++}
2. K^{+}
3. Ca^{++}
4. All.

Q.220. Plasma potassium concentration is what present of total body potassium:

1. 0.4
2. 7.6
3. 10.4
4. 89.6.

Q.221. Chromium compounds have been implicated as carcinogenic for:

1. Nasal cavity
2. Stomach
3. Lungs
4. Skin.

Q.222. Sodium content of CSF is __mg%:

1. 204
2. 264
3. 334
4. 384.

Q.223. Which of the following elements is known to influence the body's ability to handle oxidative stress ?

1. Calcium
2. Iron
3. Patassium
4. Selenium.

Q.224. Biological role of metallothioneins is to sequester harmful metal ions. These bind:

1. Cd^{++}, Cu^{++} and Zn^{++}
2. Al^{+++}, Hg^{++}, and NH_4^{+}
3. Pt^{++}, As^{+++} and PO_4^{--}
4. Fe^{+++}, Na^{+} and K^{+}.

Q.225. Total iron binding capacity, all are true except:

1. Decrease in iron deficiency anemia
2. As an direct measure of serum transferrin levels
3. Is normally one third saturated with iron
4. Will probably be reduced in nephrotic syndrome.

Q.226. Free haemoglobin in plasma is bound to:

1. Transferrin
2. Ceruloplasmin
3. Transcortin
4. Haptoglobin.

Q.227. Hemoblobin is responsible for__ % CO_2 transport in blood:

1. 40
2. 70
3. 90
4. 99.

Q.228. Chloride shift is:

1. HCO_3^- leaving the RBC in exchange of Cl^-
2. Cl^- leaving the RBC in exchange of HCO_3^-
3. H_2CO_3 leaving the RBC
4. H^+ leaving the RBC for each CO_2 that enters.

Q.229. Heme is converted to bilirubin mainly in:

1. Kidney
2. Liver
3. Spleen
4. Bone marrow.

Q.230. One unit of fresh blood raises the Hb concentratoin by:

1. 0.1 gm%
2. 1 gm%
3. 2 gm%
4. 2.2 gm%.

Q.231. Lead poisoning produces a significant increase in the urinary output of:

1. Porphobilinogen
2. ALA
3. Uroporphyrin III
4. Protoporphyrin IX.

Q.232. Analysis at pH 8.6 electrophoretic patterns of Hb isolated from the blood of patient heterozygous for the sickle cell gene would reveal how many bands ?

1. One
2. Two
3. Three
4. Four.

Q.233. Conjugated hyperbilirubinemia is seen in:

1. Gilbert's syndrome
2. Criggler Najjar syndrome type I
3. Criggler Najjar Type II
4. Dubin Johnson's syndrome.

Q.234. Patients having obstructive jaundice do not excrete this at all in urine:

1. Bilirubin
2. Glycocholate
3. Urobilinogen
4. Urate.

Q.235. When oxidative phosphorylaton is uncoupled, which one of the following actions take place ?

1. Phosphorylation of ADP accelerates
2. Phosphorylation of ADP continues but oxygen uptake stops
3. Phosphorylation of ADP stops but oxygen uptake continues
4. Oxygen uptake stops.

Q.236. The only component of the electron transport chain that is NOT firmly embedded in the inner mitochondrial membrane is:

1. Cytochrome C
2. Coenzyme Q
3. Cytochrome oxidase
4. NADH dehydrogenase.

Q.237. Which one of the following steps of electron transport is thought to be coupled to phosphorylation of ADP to form ATP ?

1. Coenzyme Q → NADH-Q reductase
2. Cytochrome C → Cytochrome reductase
3. O_2 → Cytochrome C
4. NADH → Flavoprotein.

Q.238. Cellular oxidation is inhibited by:

1. Cyanide
2. Carbon dioxide

3. Chocolate
4. Carbonated beverages.

Q.239. The presence of 2 extra pairs of electrons on the oxygen in water molecule results in:

1. Makes water a nonpolar solvent
2. Forms covalent bonds in the ice
3. Electronegative charge on water molecule
4. Electro positive charge on water molecule.

Q.240. Carbonic anhydrase in the kidney tubular cells is known to be associated with the reabsorption of:

1. Urea
2. Chloride
3. Bicarbonate ion
4. Carbohydrate.

Q.241. The most important buffer in RBC is:

1. O_2 Hb + K-hemoglobinate
2. O_2 Hb + Na-Hemoglobinate
3. $H_2CO_3 + K^+ HCO_2$
4. $H_2CO_3 + NaHCO_3$.

Q.242. A patient is suffering from untreated diabetes. His symptoms include thirst, frequent urination, weight loss, hyperventilation and fatigue. Blood analysis reveals above normal glucose levels E1 below normal bicarbonate levels, pH and pCO_2. Which one of the following conditions does this patient exhibit ?

1. Respiratory acidosis with compensatory metabolic alkalosis
2. Respiratory alkalosis with compensatory metabolic acidosis
3. Metabolic acidosis with compensatory respiratory alkalosis
4. Metabolic alkalosis with compensatory respiratory acidosis

Q.243. Basal metabolic rate:

1. Is not influenced by energy uptake
2. Increases in response to starvation
3. May decrease up to 50% during periods of starvation
4. Increases in direct proportion to daily energy expenditure.

Q.244. For diabeties:

1. The only carbohydrate that must be eliminated in the diet is surcrose
2. Fiber increases the rate at which carbohydrate is digested and absorbed
3. Not all carbohydrate foods raise blood glucose levels at the same rate because the glycemic index of all foods is not the same
4. Who are normally in good control, stress will have no effect on their blood sugar levels.

Q.245. In patients fed an equal amount (on a molar basis) of carbohydrates and fats, the respiratory quotient is:

1. 2.72
2. 1.00
3. 0.86
4. 0.70.

Q.246. Which of the following would not be included in formulating an appropriate diet for a patient recovering from renal problesms ?

1. High carbohydrate
2. High protein
3. Moderate fat
4. High fiber.

Q.247. The only route through which H^+ are eliminated from the body:

1. Lung
2. Stomach
3. Kidney
4. None.

Q.248. During starvation the non protein RCS value is close to:

1. 1
2. 0.5
3. 0.25
4. 0.75.

Q.249. Which of the following statements correctly describes allosteric enzymess:

1. Effectors may enhance or inhibit substrate binding
2. they are not usually controlled by feeback inhibition
3. The regulatory site may be the catalytic site
4. Michaelis- Menten kinetics describe their activity.

Q.250. In scurvy, post translationsal modificaton of protein fails to result in the formation of:

1. Glycoproteins
2. Tryptophan
3. Histidine
4. Hydroxyproline.

ANSWERS

1. (4)	**2.** (3)	**3.** (2)	**4.** (2)	**5.** (1)	**6.** (4)	**7.** (3)	**8.** (3)	**9.** (4)	**10.** (2)
11. (2)	**12.** (1)	**13.** (4)	**14.** (4)	**15.** (2)	**16.** (1)	**17.** (2)	**18.** (1)	**19.** (1)	**20.** (3)
21. (3)	**22.** (3)	**23.** (2)	**24.** (1)	**25.** (2)	**26.** (1)	**27.** (2)	**28.** (1)	**29.** (4)	**30.** (3)
31. (1)	**32.** (4)	**33.** (3)	**34.** (3)	**35.** (3)	**36.** (1)	**37.** (2)	**38.** (4)	**39.** (2)	**40.** (4)
41. (3)	**42.** (2)	**43.** (3)	**44.** (4)	**45.** (4)	**46.** (1)	**47.** (1)	**48.** (3)	**49.** (1)	**50.** (3)
51. (3)	**52.** (3)	**53.** (2)	**54.** (4)	**55.** (3)	**56.** (2)	**57.** (2)	**58.** (1)	**59.** (1)	**60.** (1)
61. (3)	**62.** (1)	**63.** (3)	**64.** (3)	**65.** (1)	**66.** (2)	**67.** (3)	**68.** (2)	**69.** (4)	**70.** (2)
71. (4)	**72.** (2)	**73.** (3)	**74.** (4)	**75.** (4)	**76.** (4)	**77.** (4)	**78.** (4)	**79.** (3)	**80.** (1)
81. (4)	**82.** (3)	**83.** (1)	**84.** (1)	**85.** (1)	**86.** (1)	**87.** (1)	**88.** (3)	**89.** (3)	**90.** (4)
91. (4)	**92.** (1)	**93.** (3)	**94.** (3)	**95.** (1)	**96.** (3)	**97.** (3)	**98.** (?)	**99.** (2)	**100.** (3)
101. (1)	**102.** (3)	**103.** (4)	**104.** (4)	**105.** (1)	**106.** (3)	**107.** (2)	**108.** (4)	**109.** (1)	**110.** (2)
111. (1)	**112.** (2)	**113.** (2)	**114.** (3)	**115.** (3)	**116.** (4)	**117.** (2)	**118.** (2)	**119.** (2)	**120.** (3)
121. (4)	**122.** (1)	**123.** (1)	**124.** (3)	**125.** (1)	**126.** (4)	**127.** (3)	**128.** (2)	**129.** (1)	**130.** (1)
131. (4)	**132.** (1)	**133.** (1)	**134.** (2)	**135.** (1)	**136.** (1)	**137.** (2)	**138.** (1)	**139.** (1)	**140.** (1)
141. (3)	**142.** (3)	**143.** (3)	**144.** (3)	**145.** (3)	**146.** (4)	**147.** (4)	**148.** (1)	**149.** (2)	**150.** (3)
151. (4)	**152.** (4)	**153.** (2)	**154.** (4)	**155.** (1)	**156.** (4)	**157.** (2)	**158.** (1)	**159.** (3)	**160.** (2)
161. (4)	**162.** (?)	**163.** (2)	**164.** (2)	**165.** (4)	**166.** (3)	**167.** (1)	**168.** (3)	**169.** (1)	**170.** (1)
171. (1)	**172.** (4)	**173.** (1)	**174.** (4)	**175.** (1)	**176.** (2)	**177.** (2)	**178.** (1)	**179.** (3)	**180.** (1)
181. (1)	**182.** (1)	**183.** (1)	**184.** (1)	**185.** (2)	**186.** (2)	**187.** (4)	**188.** (4)	**189.** (4)	**190.** (1)
191. (1)	**192.** (1)	**193.** (3)	**194.** (3)	**195.** (2)	**196.** (3)	**197.** (1)	**198.** (4)	**199.** (3)	**200.** (2)
201. (2)	**202.** (3)	**203.** (4)	**204.** (4)	**205.** (4)	**206.** (4)	**207.** (1)	**208.** (3)	**209.** (2)	**210.** (4)
211. (3)	**212.** (1)	**213.** (3)	**214.** (2)	**215.** (1)	**216.** (1)	**217.** (4)	**218.** (2)	**219.** (2)	**220.** (1)
221. (3)	**222.** (3)	**223.** (4)	**224.** (1)	**225.** (1)	**226.** (4)	**227.** (3)	**228.** (1)	**229.** (3)	**230.** (?)
231. (2)	**232.** (2)	**233.** (4)	**234.** (3)	**235.** (3)	**236.** (1)	**237.** (4)	**238.** (1)	**239.** (3)	**240.** (3)
241. (1)	**242.** (3)	**243.** (3)	**244.** (3)	**245.** (3)	**246.** (2)	**247.** (3)	**248.** (4)	**249.** (1)	**250.** (4)